Healing Cancer

The Top 12 Non-Toxic Cancer Treatments To Help You Beat Cancer

Simon & Enrida Kelly

Cover design by Zoe Yull (www.digican.co.uk)

Text design and typesetting by Decent Typesetting (www.decenttypesetting.co.uk)

British Library Cataloguing-in-Publication Data

A CIP record for this book is available from the British Library.

ISBN 0-95446-368-4

Disclaimer

The information in this book has been compiled from sources believed to be reliable and true. However, cancer therapy is an evolving field that is constantly being revised as new understandings are gained. Therefore, neither the authors nor the publishers can accept responsibility for errors or omissions (human or otherwise), or for any medical outcome from the use of any therapeutic strategy discussed. Readers are advised take the advice of their physician regarding the relevance and appropriateness of any particular piece of information contained in this book. The purpose of this book is to inform and the information is not intended as medical advice.

For wholesale orders please contact:

The London Press
Tel: ++44 (0)871 218 0214
Fax: ++44 (0)207 748 4424
E-mail: sales@thelondonpress.co.uk
Website: www.thelondonpress.co.uk

Website: You will find a website listing updates (and various documents referenced in this book) at www.healing-cancer.co.uk

Printed and bound by Antony Rowe Ltd, Eastbourne

Contents

Index of Interviews with Leading Professionals

Acknowledgements

Special thanks for the contribution made to this book by the following individuals (listed alphabetically by surname): Rob Barns, John Boik, Dr Stanislaw Burzynski, Marilyn Casey, Dr John Clement, Bill Dann, Peter Durden, Leonard Freeman, Roderick Howie, Sue Kelly, David King, Dr Fuad Lechin, Mark Lester, Dr Ralph Moss, Jacinte and Gaston Naessens, Dr Bill Porter, Den Rasplicka and Bill Wolcott.

A big thank you to Paul Winter for the assistance provided with the section on Cantron.

In addition, thank you to the many other friends and acquaintances who have supported and encouraged us to complete the project. This includes all those individuals we know (or have known) who have been forced to deal directly or indirectly with the illness of cancer. Your stories and experiences have stayed with us, and have become part of this book.

A thank you to Microsoft is most definitely warranted because their generous employee income protection scheme (and professional kindness) supported us during the time period our attention was first drawn to this area of research (i.e. the time during which Simon was taken seriously ill).

Lastly, but of course, by no means least, a special mention for our daughter, 'Samya the Cool-Girl Princess'.

Foreword by Etienne Callebout M.D.

Y
OU ARE ABOUT TO READ a most unusual and unique book. The authors have
sought out the foremost, most eminent individuals from around the
world, dedicated to finding solutions to cancer. What stands out for the
reader in *Healing Cancer*, is the quality of the material presented, along with the
way the book is structured—a combination of interviews with the above
mentioned medical pioneers, together with exceptionally rigorous and system-
atic explanations of their work. Personally, I would urge you to read the interviews first and then move on to the more scientifically presented material, as this
will provide depth that you will not find in other books covering this subject.

The therapies presented in the *Healing Cancer* have been meticulously
selected, with particular regard to their mode of functioning and evidence of
success. Unfortunately, up until now, these therapies have been mostly
neglected, except by the few willing to examine and challenge the prevailing
mindset and its inherent prejudices.

The medical, (albeit unconventional), practitioners featured in *Healing
Cancer* have not bowed to pressure from the big companies, who promote only
one way of thinking—and practicing medicine—and who do this via a process
of political decision-making, (which has the effect of discrediting even the initi-
ation of any alternative cancer research). In this regard, it is most likely that
Healing Cancer will alert you to other possibilities worth considering; perhaps
adding therapies to those you are already involved with.

No one has any monopoly on truth when it comes to cancer therapies; but as
abundant literature already exists on chemotherapy, radiotherapy, surgery,
hormonal treatments and so on, there is an urgent need for a book examining
the most serious complementary and unconventional, non-toxic cancer treatments. *Healing Cancer* meets this need.

Surgery and other hospital-based treatments have saved many lives and hold
irrefutable merit, but there is potential for greater success still. If only we could
integrate everything that works, irrespective of its source? Problems of egotism
(in both the mainstream and non-mainstream fields) are too often, a barrier to
progress, and therefore, the authors take us on a journey past egoism—and
sensationalism—into a sincere and honest search for accurate and responsible
information/guidance about non-toxic, unconventional cancer treatments.

Features of particular interest include the work of Dr. Lechin—a medical expert of the highest calibre—and the author of over 170 published scientific documents demonstrating efficacy of his unique and groundbreaking therapeutic approach. Yet, paradoxically, Dr Lechin is virtually unknown in the western world. In his work he has developed a way of profiling an individuals brain neurotransmitters to see whether they are of a normal or diseased profile. As neurotransmitters are, figuratively speaking, the puppet-strings of the entire body, the importance of Dr. Lechin's development of a non-invasive, non-toxic therapy capable of moving an individuals neurochemical profile from a diseased state, into a state which represents normal health, holds enormous potential for the treatment of an incalculable number of presently untreatable illnesses—cancer being number one on the list. Hopefully Dr Lechin's work will come to gain widespread renown, as it is truly unique and there is a wealth of irrefutable evidence to demonstrate its efficacy.

The contribution in *Healing Cancer* from John Boik, a research scientist at one of the world's leading cancer treatment research institutions, the MD Anderson Cancer Centre at the University of Texas is invaluable, as is that of Bill Wolcott—one of the principal developers of a system known as metabolic typing. John Boik is the first researcher to calculate the amounts and combinations of natural substances that are likely to be required to stimulate cancer cells, for example, to turn back into normal cells, while Bill Wolcott has developed a system of metabolic typing which analyses a person's metabolism to ensure that they are consuming foods (and ratios of macronutrients) that balance their system and enhance overall health.

As you will read, apart from attacking cancer directly, there are many other approaches which can be integrated. My own work has been concerned with using a wealth of new material to work out the best of these approaches, and I am pleased that this book has approached matters from a similarly holistic viewpoint. I therefore view *Healing Cancer* as an invaluable ally to the work I do in my Harley Street clinic, some fundamentals of which I will now very briefly outline, so as to introduce the reader to the concept of taking a multidimensional approach to cancer—and health in general.

The first thing in any treatment is to look at what sort of tumour/cancer we are encountering, and to examine how it interacts with the surrounding tissues. Does it, for example, secrete destructive enzymes into its immediate environment, or does it 'instruct' the body to grow blood vessels to feed it (angiogenesis). In addition, an individual's immune system must be examined to see if there are other toxins or infections – even if relatively minor – that might detract from their immune system's specific ability to counter the cancer cells. Many other factors must also be looked at, such as the eliminatory functions of the body (sweat, excrement, etc.), the person's mental state, as well as matters of nutrition, hydration and oxygenation – to name but a few. This book is important in taking into full consideration all these factors. *Healing Cancer* also appreciates that treatments of differing complexity are appropriate for each individual patient.

As stated earlier, I do not consider that any one person (or approach) has all the answers when it comes to cancer, yet still, there are too many potential solutions in danger of being ignored. *Healing Cancer* is one of the first books to bring the most important of these approaches to the attention of the public in a lucid and comprehensive way. From here, it is up to each individual to do any further research needed to collate points of view… in short to take a measure of responsibility for his or her own health.

Let us not forget either, that many conventional therapies can be used in conjunction with many of the therapies detailed in this book, as well as visa versa. Above all *Healing Cancer* demonstrates how crucial it is to think inclusively while picking a route down which to go in terms of treatment.

Dr Etienne Callebout

September 2004

Preface

IN DECEMBER OF 1999 I fell prey to a serious illness called myasthenia gravis. Myasthenia gravis is an illness in which a serious imbalance of the immune system causes the body to attack itself. Attacks are targeted at nerve signal receptor cells present on the surface of skeletal muscles throughout the body, (also known as voluntary muscles)—causing widespread chronic muscle weakness, and most characteristically, the eyelids to remain permanently closed. The illness is also known by a more descriptive name—'Rag Doll' syndrome. Only fifteen percent of individuals receiving orthodox medication experience a complete remission of the illness—eighty five percent of individuals never fully recover.[1] (Some studies indicate remission rate can be increased by removal of an individual's thymus gland but this is controversial and not proven.[2,3])

Determined to recover without the use of *steroid chemotherapy* (the usual mainstream treatment employed for myasthenia) or other potentially damaging and/or life threatening treatments, I began scouring the globe for other viable unconventional treatments. However, as I was conducting my research, I noticed many of the most promising and original therapies in the alternative health sphere were actually 'happening' around cancer. Because I had a similar interest (i.e. an immune system that was malfunctioning), as well as a general lifelong fear and lack of knowledge about cancer treatments, I decided to investigate, in depth, the various therapies I was coming into contact with.

Of course, like most people, I have known or heard about many individuals who have contracted cancer. Some managed remarkably well—a mastectomy with follow-up treatment enabled them to live a long and full life. But others had a completely different experience.

Of all the many sad and frightening experiences, one particular person stands out in my memory. His name was Trigger. A giant of a man, with shoulders the size of a bull and huge fists covered in 'knuckleduster' gold rings, Trigger lived an isolated and frighteningly lonely existence in a tiny minivan, parked in a car park, very close to where I was living myself. Trigger regularly expressed his frustration at life by getting drunk—at which times he would become violent and lash out against anybody around him.

One day, Trigger announced that he had contracted cancer. I was of course surprised and, though my feelings about him were ambiguous, I was shocked by the speed of his demise. Within a few short months, physically, apart from loose skin hanging from his skeleton, there was hardly anything of him left. Whereas before I was quite terrified of him, now I could have pushed Trigger over with a single finger without fear of retribution. Though he was receiving chemotherapy—it seemed nothing more could be done—and in a short while he was dead. This was a shocking experience and reinforced the dread in me of this terrible illness.

Considering that, statistically, so many of us will contract cancer, it is surprising how seldom it's a topic of everyday conversation. For example, what is cancer… what makes it form… how does it form… why does it act in the way it does… what other therapies have researchers proposed apart from chemotherapy, radiation and surgery… and what makes this illness so difficult to cure?

However, as my research into unconventional cancer therapies deepened, I was surprised at the amount of discussion and practical proposals about therapy that exist concerning the illness—outside of mainstream treatment centres and charities. Moreover, to my surprise, I discovered there are several specialist cancer clinics around the world offering therapies that most people have never heard of, and that are never discussed by conventional doctors. I felt compelled to learn more—and the more I learnt, the more imperative it became to publish my findings—so as to be available to people like yourself. We feel the information written in 'Healing Cancer' is also essential reading for individuals with other illnesses and also people interested in preventing the occurrence of cancer.

Of course, I have used many the therapies for my own illness, and many of the approaches have now become a way of life (e.g. Metabolic Typing and Dr Lechin's Neurotransmitter Therapy, Oxygen-Ozone Therapy and all the Group 1 Therapies (see table p.8).

As I was learning and researching, one thought kept recurring in my mind. The thought was: 'Everyone with cancer should know about this information'. That's not in any way to claim this information is a magic bullet that will enable anyone to easily cure cancer, but rather to make the point that there are a lot of worthwhile therapies around (that are not commonly known about), as well as many experienced doctors and practitioners offering services not available through standard channels. For example, from my current perspective, I would undoubtedly say that even some of the low cost therapies described in this book would have enabled Trigger to at least slow down the terrible weight loss (cachexia) he experienced (and that led to such a quick death)—and probably, would have provided a lot more benefits and/or life extension for him as well.

Today, information is available as never before. Information gives choices, and those who locate it receive the benefits. For example, take the EVA® (Ex Vivo Apoptotic) test. This is a test that can help determine how great or little an effect particular chemotherapeutic agents will have *before* they are infused into the body. As you know, chemotherapy uses very unpleasant compounds, and more often than not, several different types have to be tried before the most appropriate agent (or combination of agents) is identified. However, most often, even wealthy individuals who could easily afford the test rarely have one carried out before receiving chemotherapy—simply because they do not know, or are not informed about the test's existence. This, then, is an example of the power of information.

Therefore the aim of this book is to provide you with the best possible information—to synthesise and simplify it and to separate the wheat from the chaff. The motto all along has been as above: 'Everyone with cancer should know about this information'.

(Note: It is right for professional reasons that I clarify that my wife Enrida and I have a direct interest in (and offer to clients) several of the therapies we shall discuss in the book, as well as various items of therapeutic equipment. However, we both believe this has not influenced our impartiality in any way).

Along the way there have been discoveries beyond all expectations—for instance, Dr Lechin's neurochemical profile based strategy, John Boik's work, the availability of PDT and CLT—and at times it has been difficult to contain the excitement of the prospect of sharing this information with you. Finishing this manuscript has seemed a never-ending task; but here it is, and hopefully it will serve a good purpose.

S.J.K 14th June 2004

Healing Cancer

1

Making A Start

IS IT POSSIBLE TO HEAL THE BODY OF CANCER? Within these pages we seek to answer this most important and fundamental question with integrity and honesty. Healing Cancer presents accurate and responsible guidance on the latest and most important non-toxic cancer treatments, based upon the immense knowledge and experience generously shared by the world's leading professionals in this field. It is ideal for readers new to alternative cancer therapies, as well as those seeking information on the latest breakthroughs.

Our aim is to provide you with information that will be useful for yourself, a loved one, a friend or just someone you know of, who has been diagnosed with cancer. In this book, you will find information that can make a difference—information that will give you choices. A substantial amount of the information is new, and it is important you become familiar with it as soon as possible. Some of the other information has been available in the public domain for a while, though not in a particularly accessible format. Our aim is to present it in a format that is much more user-friendly.

Cancer is a frightening disease, all the more so because of the toxicity and severity of many of the commonly offered treatments. Because of this, we have collected together some of the world's most knowledgeable professionals on the subject of alternative and *non-toxic* cancer treatments—and have included easy-to-read interviews with each of them. The professionals interviewed are researchers, scientists, doctors and/or specialist cancer clinic managers—all with a passion and dedication to developing and practicing therapies that help heal people from cancer in a non-toxic manner.

Each professional speaks about their own area of expertise. To name a few, we have John Boik speaking about the latest research into therapy using natural compounds; Dr John Clement speaking about Immuno-Augmentive Therapy (IAT) and the experience he has gained treating thousands of individuals with cancer; the same extensive practical experience is shared by Dr Burzynski—the discoverer of a unique treatment that seems to work particularly well for brain cancers; and Dr Lechin explaining to us about the development of a recent and immensely significant therapy— the Neuroimmunomodulation Approach.

Our aim has been to ask these experts and professionals, questions you would want to ask yourself—for example, in depth questions about the therapies they offer as well as questions about their experience and the results they have obtained treating cancer. The main reason we have used the interview format, is so you can hear the answers direct 'from the horse's mouth'.

In addition to the interviews, we will discuss many other therapies (including their costs) from a balanced, unbiased point of view. There is now an enormous amount of information available in the public sphere, and it can be difficult to separate the useful out from the not so useful. Starting from scratch, sorting out this information is something that might take an individual a year or more—because it is so difficult to ascertain the truth about any particular therapy. Advocates of any particular therapy always speak so passionately and convincingly about it.

However, we have processed and structured the most useful information into an easy to use table (see p.8). By way of introducing the information in the table we can say that it is structured into three main groups: general health building therapies that form a foundation for later therapies; cancer therapies that can be carried out in your locality; and lastly, cancer therapies that require you, at least initially, to visit a specific clinic for blood tests or treatment (though all of the clinics we cover offer several months of take home supplies). We hope that you will be inspired to employ therapies from all three groups. As will become clearer later in the book, we are suggesting that you pursue a multifaceted approach, using as many different therapies from each group as possible.

Of course it is most likely you are already contemplating receiving conventional therapies such as surgery, radiation or chemotherapy. For many decades there has been extreme animosity between the two camps (conventional and alternative), with the former accusing non-mainstream researchers and practitioners of being quacks and frauds, and the latter accusing the conventional institutions of arrogantly pursuing toxic, dangerous and non-proven therapies at the expense of patient's well-being.

In many senses, unconventional cancer therapy researchers and practitioners (i.e. those working with other approaches apart from chemotherapy, radiotherapy and surgery) have now established their credibility. As we shall hear later from John Boik (one of the new generation of cancer researchers) in his institution (the world famous M.D. Anderson research centre), chemotherapy is definitely *not* a hot topic of research. Rather, as understanding about cancer cells has grown, the focus has shifted away from crude toxic unspecific therapies like chemotherapy to more subtle approaches that target the way cancer cells function.

This is only to be applauded, and in future years we can look forward to the appearance of many new mainstream cancer therapies. However, there is going to be a significant time period before these new therapies are available to the public—and of course it may turn out that hopes are not so easily realised. In the meantime, the older generation of cancer therapies are still in use—in fact, more than ever before. Also, the extreme negativity and hostility of the older generation of conventional cancer professionals towards innovative alternative therapies is still very much around. The more open-minded new generation of cancer researchers and practitioners have only just begun the job of displacing the prejudices of their elders.

Because of this, we want to encourage you to straddle the historical divide that separates surgery, chemotherapy and radiation from other unconventional options and suggest that you approach all therapies with an open mind. In helping you achieve this, we will encourage you in a number of directions. First of all, we will be recommending you obtain specific information about the chances that conventional options offer a person with your sort of cancer (see p.5). It might turn out that these are good, and you can pursue conventional avenues with confidence. However, your chances may not be so good, and it might be that you would do better investigating other unconventional therapies.

Secondly, of the three main conventional options, chemotherapy has been the most severely criticised. It is our view you are best served by becoming acquainted with the criticisms made of it, as this will enable you to better understand what you are being offered—if indeed you are offered chemotherapy. We shall therefore take a look at the subject of chemotherapy in more detail later in the book (see p.189). Our approach is to encourage you not to take sides—as in reality, both sides are likely to be of value to you.

Though we have tried to minimise any contradictory recommendations between various treatments—the fact is, as you read through the book and learn about different approaches, there will be times when one professional or therapeutic approach contradicts another. We know that some readers will not find this easy, but our approach has been to provide you with a well-rounded and comprehensive selection of cancer treatments. We feel that you should know about, and be familiar with, all of the approaches discussed in this book— we have taken out anything that is not essential reading, and moved as much information as possible to the appendices. However, in terms of any contradictions between various ways forward, naturally, you will need to use your own sense of what is the right way forward for you—in combination with independent advice, discussions with your oncologist, speaking to various clinics and practitioners, etc.

A few last points about the 'formatting' of the book. The first is to point out that we will use the words 'alternative', 'unconventional' (and sometimes complimentary) interchangeably. Actually, most of the practitioners or researchers interviewed would object to being labelled as either. This is because they do not see their therapies as 'alternatives'—but rather they consider their therapies are effective enough to be mainstream. However, we have not come up with any other way of referencing alternative, unconventional or complementary therapies—and therefore apologise in advance.

You will find that on occasions we use language that implies 'you' the reader' of this book is the person dealing with cancer—and at other times language that implies it is someone else who is experiencing the cancer. Please make allowances for this if you do not have cancer yourself—and are instead seeking to help a loved one or friend.

It has been difficult to know whether to use the term 'cancer therapy' or 'anticancer therapy', and so we have used both at different times.

Two last points, whenever costs of a therapy are mentioned, you will find it quoted in UK pounds and its equivalent in dollars. The exchange rate at the time of writing was 1 UK pound to 1.60 US dollar—and therefore this is the rate of conversion we have used.

In terms of punctuation style, especially during the interviews, you will frequently come across words and comments enclosed within square brackets. We have inserted these to provide additional information and/or clarify the point being discussed.

2

Obtaining Individualised Information

A T THIS POINT we would like to recommend that you invest some of your precious funds in obtaining an individualised report from Ralph Moss about your particular type of cancer. In making this recommendation we would like to make it quite clear that we in no way benefit financially from your ordering a report, and nor have any arrangements or deals been made about the inclusion of Ralph Moss's interview in this book in return for the recommendation.

Dr Moss's report will provide an overview of your best options from conventionally available therapies, as well as a broad assessment of your chances of success with these. The report will also explain about the most promising alternative treatments for your particular kind of cancer. We are suggesting that you order a report because unbiased and 'individualised' information about the chances of success with both conventional and unconventional therapies will be invaluable in helping you make the best possible choice of therapy.

Cancer is obviously a very serious illness and in the end, information needs to be individually tailored because some treatments work much better with certain cancers than with others (this applies to conventional and unconventional therapies). For instance, before you undergo any regimes of chemotherapy or other difficult-to-tolerate therapies, it is best that you find out how successful treatment is likely to be. Some cancers respond well to chemotherapy, others do not. Yet some oncologists still routinely give chemotherapy in instances where it might be argued that the therapy is unlikely to result in positive gains.

Ralph Moss has been providing individualised reports to individuals working to heal themselves of cancer for many years and has produced reports on hundreds of different kinds of cancer. Dr Moss's knowledge, experience and resources will ensure that you receive high quality and reliable information.

The cost of a report as of November 2004 is approximately £185-63 (converted from US price $297-00). To obtain a report you will need to call, fax or mail Dr. Moss. When you call you will need to explain your precise diagnosis along with the location of any secondary tumours (metastases), whether the report is for an adult or a child and an address where the report should be sent. The contact numbers and address are as follows:

Free brochure: 1-800-980-1234
☎: (814) 238-3369
🖷: (814) 238-5865
Mail: Cancer Decisions
      PO Box 8183
      State College, PA
      16803
      New York

Website: www.cancerdecisions.com

The most convenient way to receive your report is via email in Adobe Acrobat format.

3

Top 12 Therapy Table & Group 1 Therapies – A Solid Foundation

ABLE 1 SUMMARISES what we consider to be the most important anti-cancer therapies available to you. Group 1 contains foundation therapies and Groups 2 and 3 contain our top 12 therapies. The therapies are divided into three broad groups, so you can more easily get an idea of the cost and ease of carrying out any particular therapy. We have put a huge amount of study time and effort into deciding which therapies should be listed in the table, and also, which categories they should appear in. In the beginning our list of therapies was far longer, but we questioned each one, looked at the available evidence, read and listened to what commentators had to say—and then made a decision about whether it should appear in this final version of the table. Many times therapies have changed groups, as evidence to support them as specific cancer therapies mounted or dissipated. This was the case, for example, with oxygen-ozone therapy. Though oxygen-ozone therapy is a very commonly utilised therapy in cancer clinics around the world, nothing definitive exists to

Group	Name of therapy or approach
Group 1 Therapies [Therapies that act as a good foundation for general health & pave the way for specific cancer therapies]	1 Water/Hydration Therapy 2 Organic Food 3 Wheatgrass / Barleygrass & Spirulina Supplement 4 Mind-Body Approaches / Support Group 5 Liver Cleanse / Liver Support 6 Intestinal Cleansing / Detoxification Support 7 Wide Spectrum Nutritional Support 8 Parasite Cleanse 9 Reduce Or Eliminate Dairy Products 10 Oxygen-Ozone Therapy
Group 2 Therapies [Therapies you can carry out on a local basis in conjunction with a health professional]	1 Natural Anti-Cancer Compounds (as discussed by John Boik)* 2 Diet / Food Therapy – Metabolic Typing 3 Photodynamic Therapy* 4 Burzynski's Aminocare® A10 5 Gaston Naessen's 714-X Therapy 6 Pancreatic Enzyme supplementation 7 Cantron 8 B-17 & Hydrazine Sulphate * More experimental form of treatment. Limited data available. Should definitely be carried out in conjunction with practitioner.
Group 3 Therapies [Therapies that require you to initially visit a specialist clinic]	1 Dr Lechin's Neuroimmunomodulation Approach 2 Burzynski's Antineoplaston Therapy 3 Burton's Immuno-Augmentive Therapy 4 Photodynamic/Cellular Light Therapy (PDT/CLT)* * More experimental form of treatment. Limited data available.

*(The spine of the table reads vertically: **TOP 12 THERAPIES**)*

Table 1: Division of Therapies into the Three Main Groups

show that it causes *direct regression* of tumours. However, there is evidence suggesting it can be very beneficial to overall health—and a good chance it may help the body deal with cancer. Therefore, after taking all this into account, we have listed oxygen-ozone therapy as a Group 1 Therapy rather than a Group 2 specific anti-cancer therapy.

We have tried to provide you with a balanced list of therapies: balanced between those that cost little, and those that cost significantly more; balanced between those you can carry out at home, and those therapies that need you to visit a specialised clinic; and finally, balanced between 'naturopathic best-practice' therapies that lay a solid foundation for recovery, and those therapies that are specifically designated as anti-cancer therapies.

For instance, the first therapy listed in Group 1 Therapies is Water/Hydration Therapy. Of course it is extremely unlikely that drinking more water is going to cure cancer—but intake of sufficient quantities of high quality water is viewed as a basic prerequisite and building block of health & healing. Another way of explaining our mix of different therapies, and specifically the inclusion of Group 1 Therapies, is that if you visited a specialist cancer clinic, more than likely you would carry out many of the Group 1 Therapies as a support to your main therapy.

Broadly speaking, therapies in Group 1 are the easiest to carry out, are possible to do at home, and generally cost the least. Group 1 Therapies are not specific cancer therapies, but rather represent the fundamentals of a 'best-practice' lifestyle. They support the body in its smooth functioning, through making sure that all necessary nutrients are present, and that cleansing and detoxification processes are operating as efficiently as possible. Group 1 Therapies also address the antioxidant systems of the body and the mind-body connection (psychoimmunology). We will say a little more about each of the therapies listed in Group 1 later in this chapter.

Introducing Groups 2 and 3 (our Top 12), we can say that they are all specific anti-cancer therapies. The difference between the two groups is that it will be possible for you to carry out Group 2 Therapies either on your own, or in conjunction with a health professional in your local area, whereas in contrast, Group 3 Therapies need you to visit a specialised clinic, at least initially, for blood tests and treatment. However, all Group 3 Therapies are possible to carry out at home after initial visits to the clinics. In general, Group 3 Therapies are likely to be higher cost therapies, especially when travel and accommodation are taken into account.

We should note that Group 3 Therapies are some of the most powerful choices you have available to overcome cancer and accordingly it is our hope you will plan and spread your budget over all three groups. This would mean you incorporate many of the Group 1 Therapies into your everyday lifestyle; that you carry out several of the Group 2 Therapies locally or at home, and that you also make a visit to at least one of the specialised clinics.

It is our view that this is your best way to proceed as it represents a truly multi-tiered approach to cancer—built on the foundation of a 'best-practice' lifestyle. You might already be receiving, or intending to undergo, conventional therapies as well—and there is no reason why you cannot combine the two approaches. There is good evidence to suggest that many of the unconventional therapies covered in this book support and enhance the effects of conventional therapies.

Our concern is that this may seem a bit complicated for you. However, we would like to assure you that all this is easier and more enjoyable than you might at first anticipate. We encourage you to start slowly and incorporate one new therapy every few days. Proceeding one step at a time will prevent you from becoming overloaded—and give you time to research Group 3 Therapies in more depth.

Of course monies are likely to be an issue for most people, so it is best that we briefly discuss this issue. Certainly in the UK, any medical treatment that we receive through the National Health Service (NHS) is free of charge—and we are not used to putting any of our own monies towards health care costs. However, quite a lot of people do spend an increasing amount on health supplements such as vitamins and minerals, and private health care plans are becoming increasingly popular, especially as part of a job benefits package. But the bottom line, is that spending our own monies on health care is not something we usually do here in the UK. Traditionally, savings go towards a summer holiday, a new car or an extension to the house. We might even suggest that the culture in the UK is such that spending money on health care is seen as unnecessary, when care can be obtained free of charge. We encourage you to take the opposite view, and consider any monies put towards your health as an investment in your future. Of course there are no guarantees—but surely you or your loved one deserve to be able to utilise the very best.

Certainly the clinics we have listed that offer Group 3 Therapies won't take your money unless they feel you stand a reasonable chance of improvement. Before you even visit, a doctor from the clinic will need to speak with you on the telephone to find out how you are, what type of cancer you are dealing with, what treatments you have already received (conventional and/or unconventional), how able you are to travel, etc. From this information, together with their experience, they will be able to indicate whether they might be able to help.

With regard to private health plans, there is a good chance—as you would expect—that they will refuse to cover the costs of unconventional therapies.

There have, nonetheless, been several court cases in the US in which courts have ordered health insurance companies to pay for Burzynski's Antineoplaston treatment. The courts deemed, even though the medical community doesn't officially sanction the therapy, the evidence indicates that for certain cancers, antineoplastons are as likely to be effective as other conventionally accepted treatments. Therefore, there is no reason for health insurance companies to refuse to cover the costs of treatment. The lesson from this is to push hard, and at least try to make your insurance company pay.

One other source of funding could be friends or relatives. It is easy to dismiss this approach because none of us like to ask for money, but as you will see, the amount you will need to raise to visit one of the Group 3 clinics is not outrageous. Also, because cancer is such a frightening illness (and so many of us are likely to be affected by it), our feeling is that most people are happy to contribute—even if it is just to see whether the therapy is worth pursuing in the event they themselves contract cancer. With regard to monies, Anne and David Frähm, authors of 'A Cancer Battle Plan', make the point that sending a cheque to someone struggling with cancer is one of the most useful and valuable ways to help.[1]

Finding a therapist: We have mentioned, several times, the importance of locating an experienced therapist. As in all undertakings in life, sometimes the going gets tough, and you will need a confident and strong guiding hand to see you over any rocky patches. We also recommend you place yourself under the supervision of a medical doctor who can monitor your progress. (See www.acam.org or www.ompress.com for some listings of worldwide medical doctors with an interest in emerging unconventional therapies).

At the same time, don't let a therapist or doctor make your decisions for you, or limit you to a certain course of action. Working with a health professional is a two-way partnership, and together you need to form a close and respectful working alliance. Let your feelings be your guide in this. If you don't feel right about a certain professional, then trust your feelings, and locate another one.

Locating a therapist for Group 1 Therapies is not necessarily an imperative. They are all very simple therapies and can be easily incorporated into your everyday life. To help you do this, we will provide a brief overview of each of the therapies listed under Group 1. Where possible, we will also indicate approximate costs.

Here we should note that the one item we have missed off the Group 1 listing is sunlight. This is because conventional medical advice seems to be for us to avoid sunlight as much as possible (or at least cover ourselves in UV blocking cream). However, in the naturopathic field, morning and late afternoon levels of sunlight are viewed as necessary to health (approx twenty minutes a day on as

Description of therapy	Cost/day	Cost/month
Hydration Therapy	£1.00	£30.00
Organic Food	Slightly more than present food bill	
Wheatgrass / Barleygrass / Spirulina	£0.75	£22.50
Mind.Body Approaches / Support Group	Locate free weekly support group	
Liver Cleanse / Liver Support	Virtually no cost	
Intestinal Cleansing / Detoxification Support	£0.30	£9.00
Wide Spectrum Nutritional Support	£2.20	£66.00
Parasite Cleanse	£0.50/day for month. Total £15.00	
Reduce Or Eliminate Dairy Products	No cost	
Ozone Therapy (two sessions per week)	£10.00	£300.00
Total without including Ozone Therapy	£4.75	£142.50
Total with inclusion of Ozone Therapy	£14.75	£442.00

Table 2: Breakdown of Group 1 Therapy Costs in UK Pounds

much of the body as possible).[2] You will be able to read about the possible connection of sunlight to staying free of cancer in the section on (p.146).

If you are interested in finding out more about the clinically demonstrated benefits of sensible sun exposure on bone, cellular, organ, autoimmune and mood-related health, please see The UV Advantage, by Dr Michael F. Holick of the Boston University School of Medicine. (Published by: Simon & Schuster, ISBN: 0743486471.)

Group 1 Therapies

Approximate cost is between £4-75 ($7.60) & £14-75 ($23-60) per day.

INTRODUCTION: The approximate daily cost of Group 1 Therapies is £4.75 ($7.60) without oxygen-ozone therapy, and £14.75 ($23.60) with oxygen-ozone therapy. This figure is based on locating a free support group, rather than one that you would have to pay for. Also we have omitted the small one-off charges

Description of therapy	Cost/day	Cost/month
Hydration Therapy	$1.60	$48.00
Organic Food	Slightly more than present food bill	
Wheatgrass / Barleygrass / Spirulina	$1.20	$36.00
Mind.Body Approaches / Support Group	Locate free weekly support group	
Liver Cleanse / Liver Support	Virtually no cost	
Intestinal Cleansing / Detoxification Support	$0.48	$14.40
Wide Spectrum Nutritional Support	$3.52	$105.60
Parasite Cleanse	$0.80/day for month. Total $24.00	
Reduce Or Eliminate Dairy Products	No cost	
Ozone Therapy (two sessions per week)	$16.00	$480.00
Total without including Ozone Therapy	**$7.60**	**$228.00**
Total with inclusion of Ozone Therapy	**$23.60**	**$707.20**

Table 3: Breakdown of Group 1 Therapy Costs in US Dollars

for an enema kit, hypnotherapy relaxation tape or the very small costs of doing a liver cleanse.

As you can see, without ozone therapy the very approximate costs of carrying out Group 1 Therapies are £142.50 ($228.00) per month. By including ozone therapy, the cost is significantly increased, though we should note that ozone therapy is a therapeutic modality in itself (i.e. it is something more than foundational support—more explanation later). With ozone therapy the cost per month rises to around £442.00 ($707.20).

With regard to the costs of ozone therapy that we have supplied so far, we should note that these are based upon receiving the therapy at a practice or clinic. However, ozone therapy is one of the therapies where it makes economic sense to own your own equipment, though you should always receive a number of sessions from a skilled practitioner first. (The costs of purchasing ozone therapy equipment will be detailed in a later section.)

Now that we have an outline of Group 1 Therapies and costs, we will look at each Group 1 Therapy in a little more detail.

Water/Hydration Therapy

Approx cost: £1.00 per day (Glass bottles)

This is first on the list because there is no reason not to drink 1.5–2 litres of good quality water every day. Water has been described as one of the most universal solvents on the planet, and is used both for hydrating the trillions of cells that make up your body and for dissolving toxic waste substances so that they can be efficiently excreted out of your system.

The best water is fresh unpolluted spring water. However, not many of us have access to this, so in its place a good-tasting still water is sufficient. If you have the funds, glass bottles are better than plastic (there is no leeching of plastic residues into the water). Tap water is *not* recommended, unless it has gone through a high quality filtration system.

Organic Food

Approx cost: Cutting down on processed food can easily pay for the extra costs of organic food

We are sure you do not need us to go through the benefits of organic food. Apart from the fact animals and plants are treated with more respect, many studies have documented factory farmed produce to be of inferior quality in terms of vitamins, minerals and other important nutrients not to mention the possibly dangerous and environmentally destructive pesticides they contain.[3]

Many people are put off by the extra cost of organic produce. However, it is actually processed foods that are exorbitant in their cost—not organic foods. By cutting down on 'ready-made' meals and switching to a more wholesome 'basic' diet, you will find you save money by eating organic.

Also, in our opinion, organically produced food often tastes better than intensively produced food. This can be verified by the simplest of scientific experiments—comparing the taste, for example, of an organic egg with a factory farmed egg or an intensively grown potato with an organic potato. Though there are bound to be exceptions, we are sure you will find organic generally tastes far better.

As we will see in the section on Metabolic Typing, food is one of the most powerful 'medicines' you can use. Metabolic Typing will help you identify the 'right' kind of food for your type—and eating organic will ensure the 'medicine' is of the highest possible quality.

Wheatgrass / Barleygrass & Spirulina Supplement

Approx cost: £0.75 per day

This is a low priced supplement in health shops—though if you have the time and inclination some say it is better to grow wheatgrass or barleygrass at home and then freshly juice it. However, you probably have much better things to be getting on with, and a supplement is fine, especially if it is organic.

Wheatgrass and barleygrass are considered to be two of the most nutritious substances that grow on the earth, and they contain a whole spectrum of vitamins and minerals—all in an easily absorbable form. Some practitioners consider wheatgrass therapy to be an important cancer therapy in its own right.[4]

Further, considering the recent breakthrough in understanding of the role that chlorophyll and sunlight appear to play in the human body (see p.146), it would seem a wise move to increase your intake of chlorophyll rich substances. For instance, spirulina supplements are useful in this regard as they are high in available chlorophyll—though, as you will read, sunlight is an important part of the equation as well.

Mind-Body Approaches

Hypnosis/Relaxation Tape – approx cost: £10.00 (once-off)
Therapy/Support Group – approx cost: Nil – £30.00 per week

Interestingly, studies have indicated that individuals who are a member of a well-run support group live twice as long as those who are not a member of such a group.[5]

The psychological and spiritual aspect of your illness is a very important part and demands as much attention as the physical part. Illness is often a transformational time—a time when you may change direction in your life.

Making use of this space and transformational time could well be an important factor in generating an improvement in your health. Dr Patrick Donovan, for example, views the 'chaos of cancer' as part of a process of change and transformation in a person's way of being, and believes that resources should be directed to supporting and making sense of this.[6] So join a therapy or support group… though it can be daunting at first, it can be a very worthwhile and profound experience. Another option is to find a therapist for one to one counselling. This too can be an extremely rewarding experience and you are likely to feel surprised at just how healing exploring various emotions and thoughts can be. We recommend you locate a 'Person Centred' counsellor, as this form of therapy will not attempt to fit you into any particular 'theoretical framework', but will approach you as a completely unique individual. If funds are an issue, you are likely to be able to obtain lower cost therapy through a counselling college in your locality.

Also, purchase a hypnotic tape to help you relax and eliminate stress. Hypnotic tapes are enjoyable to listen to and very relaxing. The body heals best when it is relaxed, and also of great importance, when it is obtaining sufficient hours of deep sleep. During sleep you should reach the stage of 'slow wave sleep' (SWS), which is the deepest level of sleep (and deeper than REM dreaming sleep). Various products, such as magnetic pillows and sleep inducing 'music' are available for purchase through many outlets on the internet. Objective investigations and/or reviews of these products are rare and usually superficial, but do however oftentimes indicate therapeutic value.

Liver Cleanse / Liver Support

Approx cost: £1.00 per time (carry out three times in total, once every two to three weeks)

Within the naturopathic field, the liver cleanse is considered to be a most valuable and useful therapy. It is also one of the lowest cost therapies listed in the table. Your liver is responsible for carrying out hundreds of essential chemical processes and its optimum functioning is vital for proper metabolism and detoxification. The liver cleanse is a simple procedure that takes about thirty hours from beginning to end. It will cost you virtually nothing, and hopefully you will have improved liver functioning after two or three treatments.

Many people report eliminating hundreds of stones after carrying out the cleanse, and it would seem that these stones are not gall stones, but are stones formed from cholesterol that then 'sit' in the bile ducts contained within the liver, clogging it and impeding its function. You will find instructions about how to carry out the cleanse in the appendices, along with some website references where you can view pictures of the type and number of stones that individuals have excreted during the procedure. The pictures are quite remarkable and well worth a look. (Please note: You should always carry out a liver flush in conjunction with a health professional.)

Intestinal Cleansing / Detox Support

Reusable Enema Kit approx cost: £10.00
Ground Flax (Linseed) or Psyllium Husks approx cost: £0.30 per day

It is important your digestive system is functioning correctly. The naturopathic approach considers that both health and disease originate in the colon. Faeces should move constantly and be eliminated quickly and regularly. It is generally agreed humans should eliminate faeces twice a day and that stools should be well formed. You will know if you have regular bowel movements and therefore, whether your colon is in good health. Naturopathy considers that disease originates in the colon, because when colon functioning is poor it allows highly toxic waste material to build up and be absorbed by the body.

If you feel your colon needs attention, you might want to consider a course of colonic irrigation sessions (around £75 each), as these are considered the best way to cleanse the whole colon. Then, longer term, you can treat yourself regularly using a simple enema kit.

A question often asked is whether colonic irrigation, or an enema, is a safe and healthy procedure, especially in terms of maintaining the 'intestinal flora' (micro organisms such as lactobacillus that inhabit the intestine). In answer, we can state that enemas are considered very safe even if carried out on a regular basis, because generally they only wash the lowest part of the colon and rectum. Of great importance is the fact that this is the area where 70% of bowel/colon cancers develop.[7] On the other hand, colonic irrigation, which washes the whole colon much more thoroughly, should be carried out for just four – six sessions (on a weekly basis)—with a possible follow-up session around six weeks later.

It is of note that the Gerson program (a well known cancer program advocating the consumption of large quantities of fruit and vegetable juice to obtain high levels of nutrients) recommends regular coffee enemas (the coffee being cool of course) to help the body detoxify. The reason being that coffee, when taken into the colon, causes the liver to release stored toxins into the intestine where they can easily be excreted from the body. In many ways, a coffee enema has a similar function to the liver cleanse described above, though it can be done more often than every three weeks. Coffee also contains anti-cancer substances and these are best absorbed when coffee is infused into the colon, rather than when it is drunk.[8] Please see the appendices for details on how to perform a coffee enema.

A final point: for most of history, colonic irrigation and/or enemas have been the preserve of nobles, the rich, and in present times, film stars and celebrities. They have so valued the procedure because they know from experience how much it supports health and helps them to stay looking young and beautiful. It is hoped this observation will cast a more favourable light on the procedure for you. To locate a therapist, contact a relevant professional association or register of colon hydrotherapists covering your country. As usual these days, the best place to begin is with a search on the internet.

Additional methods of improving colon health:

If you regularly experience constipation, take a preparation containing ground flax seeds or psyllium husks. (Please note: flax seeds are the better of the two as they also contain other cancer fighting compounds. Flax seeds must be ground up to obtain maximum benefit, though it is cheaper to grind up your own seeds in a coffee grinder.) Ground flax seeds and/or psyllium husks are wonder preparations. Both contain soft fibre that, when mixed with water, becomes a slippery gel able to lubricate the inner surfaces of the colon. In addition, fibre helps deal with toxic compounds produced in the colon during its normal functioning—this is why many studies have demonstrated the incidence of colon cancer is reduced by the presence of adequate fibre in the diet.

Here it is worth noting, a common misconception about 'fibre'. Most people have the impression that fibre is only a rough friction-causing substance, like coconut matting or sandpaper. Its name definitely does give this impression. However, as described, ground flax and psyllium husks contain a soft, water-soluble form of fibre which absorb around twenty times their own weight in water, making them a bulking agent as well as a lubricant.

If you regularly feel sore or itchy around you anus, it could be you are prone to constipation—or it could be you are eating or drinking something you are intolerant/allergic to. It is important you clear up this irritation because it will be preventing your colon from absorbing the nutrients your body needs. Constant inflammation is never good in any part of the body—long term it can lead to all sorts of health problems.

There are two main ways of identifying possible food intolerances. First is to consider what you are eating, and see if you can identify a food that might be causing the reaction. When you have identified a possible culprit, try eliminating it for a period of time (e.g. for two to three weeks) to see if the irritation disappears. Chances are, in most cases, it will be something very obvious that you are consuming every day (ironically, it is probably something you really crave).

Secondly, you could have a food intolerance test carried out by a reputable company. We recommend you have a laboratory blood based food intolerance test carried out rather than an electronic/frequency one. In our opinion, blood-based laboratory tests are far more accurate. Electronic allergy tests, though a promise for the future, are at present something of a 'black art' to administer—and it is not clear how accurate they are.

If you have the funds, a food intolerance test is a good idea regardless of any direct symptoms. There are many reported experiences of individuals identifying common food substances as the cause of many years discomfort and suffering. Full spectrum tests (i.e. over one hundred foods) cost around the £218 ($349) mark, though some company's offer a lower cost initial non-specific food intolerance test (i.e. the test indicates if a food intolerance is present—but does not identify the food), which you can use in the first instance to assess if the more detailed test is required. A non-specific food intolerance test is £37.00 ($59.00). See www.yorkallergyusa.com for details about how to obtain both tests.

Lastly, we should note the value of chlorophyll as a substance able to neutralise toxic substances in the stomach, intestines and colon. Toxic substances (such as heterocyclic amines—substances produced through the normal process of digestion) cause damage to DNA, and it is estimated that even a healthy human cell receives between five to ten thousand hits to their DNA each day. Most often, DNA damage is repaired by special elements within each cell (see section starting p.34 for details)—however, damage may not always be properly repaired, and DNA damage may build up to a point where a cell starts to malfunction and behave in a cancerous way. Chlorophyll and stabilised chlorophyll (chorophyllin) are recommended as substances which can significantly limit the damage toxic substances are able to inflict upon cellular DNA.[9]

Chlorophyll is a remarkable substance and is sometimes described as the 'blood' of the plant world. Comparing the molecular structure of haemoglobin with the molecular structure of chlorophyll, we find they are near identical, the main difference being that haemoglobin has a molecule of iron at its centre, while chlorophyll has a molecule of magnesium (hence the red colour of blood and the green colour of plants). In the diagram below, heme (the oxygen carry component of haemoglobin) is on the left, and chlorophyll is on the right. As you will note, both heme and chlorophyll function as 'harvesters' of oxygen.

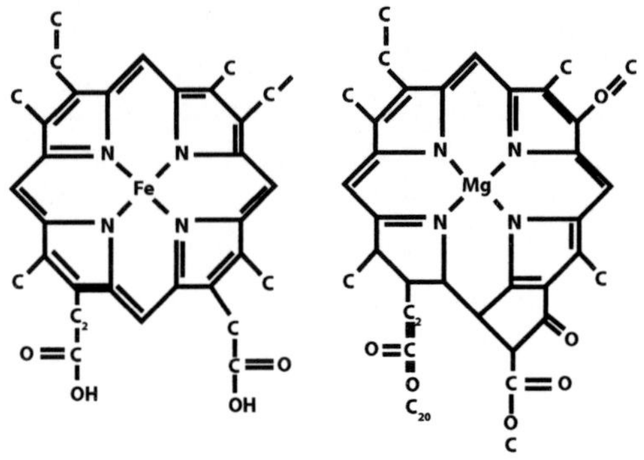

Figure 1: Comparison of heme (on left) from blood & chlorophyll

Though not specifically related to cancer, one of the most powerful demonstrations of chlorophyll's beneficial action in the body is the way it functions as an 'internal deodorant' and yeast suppressant. This is most impressive to witness, as its effects can begin after as short a period as twenty-four hours. Individuals who have suffered odour problems of the body or breath for years can find their symptoms disappear in a matter of hours. Also, in terms of therapeutic usefulness, as we have already mentioned chlorophyll is the basis of PDT/CLT—one of the new and upcoming therapies we cover in this book (see p.75 and p.146).

Nutritional Supplementation

Wide spectrum nutritional supplement – approx cost: £1.10 per day
Glutathione precursors – approx cost: £0.60 per day
Oil supplementation – approx cost: £0.50 per day

Wide spectrum nutritional supplementation

We should note there is a cross-over between nutrients we will discuss in this section, and some of natural compounds we will be examining in the section 'Natural Anti-Tumour Compounds Discussed By John Boik' (p.34). At this point however, we are just ensuring you are providing your body with the wide spectrum nutrients it needs for basic health.

There are many broad-spectrum nutrient mixes available on the market. Our favourite is the Life Extension Mix, which contains over a hundred different and vital nutrients (see www.lef.org for details).

Glutathione precursors

We need to mention the value of glutathione to optimal functioning of the human body. Its importance and value is reflected in the fact that during the last five years, over twenty-five thousand medical articles looking into its functioning have been published.[10] Glutathione is an essential substance that needs to be present in adequate quantities within each individual cell for maximum health. Its function includes donating electrons to other anti-oxidants such as vitamin C, vitamin E and lipoic acid so that these can be recycled and put back to work, as well as being an important anti-oxidant itself. It is of note, the liver (the main organ of detoxification) is the largest user of glutathione.

Even though oral glutathione and the widely available compound N-Acetyl Cysteine (NAC) are both often prescribed to increase glutathione levels (see p.202 for appropriate amounts), in fact oral glutathione does not lead to a significant increase in cellular glutathione levels, and NAC can cause undesirable side effects. A far better, safer and more efficient method of raising glutathione levels is to use specially manufactured whey protein isolates such as Immunocal or ImmunePro. On this subject, holistic practitioner Duncan Crow writes:

> 'More than 90% of glutathione taken orally gets digested [and destroyed]. The 8–10% that enters the bloodstream does not enter the cells where it is needed. Taken intravenously, it still does not enter the cells. Given as a spray, glutathione can be absorbed through sinus and lung tissue, but this is only useful for lung and sinus problems and the glutathione does not get distributed around the body.

> By far the best method of raising cellular glutathione levels is to take cold-processed whey isolate (as this contains glutathione precursors which can then be used within each cell for the manufacture of glutathione)... Second best is N-Acetyl Cysteine (NAC), which has a half life in the body of two hours, so it has to be taken every four to five hours or glutathione levels plummet, often to below original levels.

> Both oral glutathione and NAC do lead to an increase of glutathione inside the cells, but with the oral glutathione route, the increase is insignificant and NAC can have toxicity issues. NAC can cause side effects at doses of just 300mg × five per day, so is not particularly useful as a supplement but is more suitable for use as an emergency preparation.

Take glutathione increasing supplements with selenium (200–800 mcg daily) for best effect.

Dr. Jimmy Gutman's book Glutathione: The Body's Most Powerful Healing Agent, is a good medical reference on the subject, complete with peer-reviewed references. It is of note that Gutman doesn't recommend NAC at all'.[xi]

If you are intolerant to dairy products, products containing whey products such as Immunocal may not be suitable, even though they contain far lower amounts of the common intolerance causing factors (i.e. casein, fats and lactose). See Appendix C: Useful Contacts & Resources for some links to studies on cancer and glutathione as well as a small downloadable ebook with information from Gutman's book mentioned above.

Linseed / Flaxseed Oil + Fish Oil

This is another aspect of nutrition that will be repeated again in the section on Natural Anti-Tumour Compounds (p.34). Certain oils and fats (which come under the umbrella term of EFAs—essential fatty acids) are vital to health, and there are a number of different types required by the human body. Probably your best bet is to get one of the 'multi-oil' mixes that are around such as Udo's Choice.

A couple of the most important oils, in relation to cancer are flax oil and fish oil. Both are sources of EFAs (Essential Fatty Acids) which are compounds that can induce therapeutic benefits for a person with cancer. One particular point about another of flax oils major constituents, alpha linolenic acid (ALA), is worth noting. It is thought that cancer occurs so rarely in the small intestine because significant amounts of linolenic acid are naturally secreted in this part of the body.[12]

According to Joanna Budwig, for maximum effectiveness flax oil should be mixed up with a very low fat cheese called Quark (commonly available in supermarkets). Budwig explains that when it is mixed with a protein source such as Quark, flax oil becomes water soluble, and is thus able to travel through microfine capillaries to areas where it is needed. Other unsaturated oils such as olive oil are water-soluble, but to a much lesser degree.

Joanna Budwig uses flax oil as a specific therapy for people who are in the late stages of terminal cancer, and reports considerable success. Budwig reports carrying out flax oil enemas, and notes that her patients report a tremendous feeling of well-being after the proceedure.[13] Also studies investigating levels of ALA in breast cancer patients have noted that low levels appeared to be one of the most important factors that contribute to the spread of the cancer.[14]

It is generally considered that only a small amount of flax oil per day is required (two teaspoons), and it should *never* be used to cook with (it is unstable and produces many free radical compounds—always use coconut oil for cooking). Boik estimates the amount of fish oil (when used synergistically with other compounds) needed to have a therapeutic effect is in the region of six to twenty-one grams per day (see section starting p.34).

Parasite Cleanse

Approx cost: £0.50 per day

Parasites can cause many health problems, and when present, 'steal' vital nutrients from the body for their own use. It is good naturopathic practice, if chronic illness is being experienced, to take just one course of an anti-parasitic herbal formula—in case parasitic infection is present. There are several anti-parasitic formulas available and they should be taken for a four-week period. An appropriate formulation will contain ingredients such as wormwood, green hulls of black walnut, cloves, citrucidal, garlic and goldenseal. With regard to staying free of parasites—measures such as cleaning work tops with appropriately diluted hydrogen peroxide, and keeping pets away from bedding and food preparation areas are important.

Reduce or Eliminate Cows' Milk Products

Approx cost: Nil

Jane Plant has speculated a possible link between breast cancer and milk products, after her own experience of breast cancer completely healing after she eliminated milk products from her diet. We should note, however, that the link between cancer and dairy products has not been proven—though within the naturopathic world, cows' milk products have long been a cause for concern. First of all they are mucus causing, which indicates that they are irritating the body, and secondly, they contain insulin growth factor IGF-1, oestrogen and prolactin—hormones that can stimulate cells to divide and are thought to play a role in the progression of cancer.

Our advice is to cut down consumption of cows' milk products as much as possible, especially if you notice they are mucus forming. There are substitutes such as almond milk, oatmilk or rice milk, which make a good replacement. (Soymilk is not recommended as it contains oestrogen hormone, which may stimulate oestrogen dependant tumours, and cause food intolerances for many people).

Oxygen-Ozone Therapy

Approx cost: (for two sauna sessions per week) £10.00 ($16) per day, i.e. £35 ($56) per session

Ozone is produced by energising oxygen molecules so that they join together in groups of 'three' rather than in groups of 'two'—as they do when they form stable atmospheric oxygen (i.e. O_2). The gas mixture produced by a typical ozone generator generally contains around 98 to 99 percent stable oxygen (O_2) and 1–2% ozone (O_3). Both gases are oxidants, though ozone is far more reactive than oxygen, and a more powerful oxidiser. This gas mixture is then used therapeutically in a variety of ways to produce physiological improvements.

The benefits of oxygen-ozone therapy are broad and deep—two of the most important being an ability to boost immune system functioning as well as improving cellular *anti*-oxidant functioning. Bocci describes this therapeutic 'ability' as 'therapeutic shock', though we prefer the term 'therapeutic stimulation'.[15] By applying calculated and precise dosages of oxygen-ozone gas, it is possible to send a limited and controlled oxidative pulse running through an organism, which in turn promotes various beneficial effects.

Using an analogy—'therapeutic shock' or 'therapeutic stimulation' works in the same way as a pacemaker. In the same way that a pacemaker provides gentle 'electric stimulation' to keep a heart beating, oxygen-ozone 'therapeutic stimulation' reactivates aspects of cellular functioning that have become frozen or paralysed—such as the paralysis of antioxidant functionality in a person experiencing chronic oxidative stress. (Chronic oxidative stress refers to a state that occurs when an individual's anti-oxidant system is not fully functioning and not able to keep up with the continuous oxidative assaults against the body. By analogy, we could say cells existing in a state of chronic oxidative stress are likely to rust like a piece of untreated steel).

The irony therefore, of oxygen-ozone therapy, is that though oxygen-ozone gas is an oxidant, when carried out with the correct therapeutic doses, it can help an individual overcome a state of chronic oxidative stress and improve overall health. As mentioned, Bocci considers this is because the oxidative 'therapeutic stimulation' provided by the therapy is an acute, transient pulse, rather than a continual 'chronic' background stress.[16]

During the therapy, as the oxygen ozone mix comes into contact with the body, it causes an intense production of oxidised products (products formed when compounds in the body come into contact with oxygen or other oxidising agents). These products circulate around the body and act as chemical messengers, setting off a whole cascade of beneficial cellular processes (such as the immune system stimulation and increase in antioxidant functioning mentioned above). In effect, the positive processes begun in the body by the transient pulse of oxidative products seems to significantly outweigh the usual negative effects produced by oxidative stress.

It is important to note that the development of many degenerative diseases, including cancer, can be correlated with a state of chronic oxidative stress, and reducing oxidative stress is therefore a therapeutic goal worth pursuing (see discussion with Boik p.34). Specifically in regard to cancer, it is important to stimulate 'body-wide' cellular anti-oxidant functioning and lower the levels of background chronic oxidative stress—because high oxidative stress may be associated with increased DNA damage and cellular mutations—both contributing factors to the formation of cancer. (Note that chemotherapy and radiation both increase oxidative stress). The benefits of stimulating the immune system through ozone therapy are self-explanatory.

There are several different methods of therapeutically applying oxygen-ozone gas, the simplest being an oxygen-ozone steam sauna. This is also the method you are most likely to find available on a local basis—as well as the most affordable way of utilising oxygen-ozone therapy. It involves you sitting inside a sealed cabinet (just your body, arms and legs—not your head), while a mixture of steam, oxygen and ozone is introduced into the cabinet.

Steam is used in the cabinet to help the oxygen-ozone gas to make better contact with body tissues. Bocci suggests that the oxidised products formed by the action of oxygen-ozone on the surface of the skin, travel down through the tissues and into the bloodstream—and in this way provide the 'body-wide' controlled 'therapeutic stimulation'. The therapy temporarily increases blood oxygenation as well as utilising ozone's anti-bacterial, anti-viral and anti-fungal properties.

The steam cabinet method of ozone therapy has another advantage, in that it raises overall body temperature. Raising body temperature ('systemic hyper-thermia') is used as a cancer therapy in its own right at many clinics. Tumours do not tolerate heat well primarily because they are a relatively disordered mass of cells, clumped very tightly together, and are therefore not able to dissipate heat efficiently. It is generally considered that a body temperature of one hundred and four degrees Fahrenheit is detrimental to tumours.[17]

(Note: Another important heat therapy is known as Coley's Toxin's. This is a special formulation made from the toxins left over from a particular strain of dead bacteria that trigger very high temperatures when injected. The main effect of the bacterial toxins and the resulting high body temperature is to massively stimulate the immune system. The resulting immune stimulation has

even been documented to cause complete regressions of cancer. A clinic specialising in this therapy is the Issels Treatment Center in Mexico – www.issels.com).

In addition to ozone sauna therapy, there are some doctors who offer what
is known as autohemotherapy. Autohemotherapy involves removing a small
quantity of blood, mixing it with a measured quantity of ozone and then re-
infusing it back into the body. Ozonating a small amount of blood and rein-
troducing it in this way causes the same controlled 'therapeutic stimulation' we
discussed earlier. It is also possible to directly inject tumours with oxygen-
ozone gas.

Though a very common anti-cancer therapy around the world, oxygen-
ozone therapy is nevertheless a very controversial one, and it is right we attempt
to clarify both what *has* been demonstrated in studies, and what has *not* been
demonstrated. For many proponents of oxygenation therapy the theoretical
underpinning for the use of oxygen-ozone therapy against cancer is provided by
the theories of Otto Warburg (see p.231). Based on Warburg's theories (i.e. that
cancer forms as a cellular reaction to a lack of oxygen), the aim is to flood the
body with plentiful oxygen, to ensure cells have sufficient oxygen available for
efficient cellular respiration to take place (i.e. cells are able to generate energy by
using oxygen to 'burn' carbohydrates).

With direct reference to Otto Warburg's theory, we should note that Warburg
did not discuss the role of ozone in cellular processes and/or cancer—rather he
discussed the role of oxygen. Secondly, bearing in mind that oxygen-ozone
therapy uses approximately ninety eight percent oxygen, it might be expected
that oxygen-ozone therapy would cause tumours to immediately regress. That
said, reports of this happening, though numerous and very impressive to read,
are anecdotal (i.e. verbally reported) and no studies have confirmed it has this
action in-vivo (i.e. in the body).

There have been some test tube studies that have shown direct action against
cancerous cells by ozone—however we should note there is a lot of difference
between test tube studies (in-vitro) and real life actions (in-vivo).[18] For
instance, while it is easy to obtain a high concentration of ozone gas around
cancer cells in a test tube, it is difficult to achieve this in the body as ozone
breaks down instantaneously when it comes into contact with body tissues—
(direct injections of ozone into tumours are probably the only way for ozone to
make direct contact with cancerous cells).

However, as we have discussed, what *has* been documented in preliminary
studies is that oxygen-ozone therapy acts as a powerful stimulus to the body's
antioxidant system. Furthermore, in terms of cancer, oxygen-ozone therapy has
shown itself (in various studies) to beneficially modulate (i.e. balance) the
immune system, lessen the side effects of conventional cancer treatments, and

to affect a better outcome of conventional cancer treatments.[19] Studies have also shown oxygen-ozone therapy to be an effective analgesic (pain killer).[20] Here are some abstracts from various oxygen-ozone therapy studies, to give you a flavour of the kind of benefit it can have:

Ozone Therapy in a Complex Treatment of Breast Cancer (Claudia N. Kontorshchikova et al).

Involvement of ozone therapy in a complex treatment of patients with breast cancer helped to diminish the incidence and degree of cytostatic toxic side effects [inhibition or suppression of normal cellular growth and multiplication], improve their life quality and immunological parameters, and significantly increase the activity of the antioxidant defense system.

Ozone as a Modulator of the Immune System (Alessandra Larini et al)

Results show that ozone can act as a weak inducer of cytokines [immune system hormones] producing IL-6, IL-4, TNF-α, IFN-γ, IL-2 and IL-10 and, most importantly, there is a significant relationship between cytokine production and ozone concentration.

Medical Ozone for Prophylaxis and Treatment of Complications associated by Chemotherapy of Ovary Cancer (Guennadi O. Gretchkanevl et al)

The present investigation resulted in the following:

1   Ozone therapy caused an improvement in patients' state, in their sleep and appetite, and a decrease in nausea and vomiting.

2   Ozone therapy produced an immunomodulating effect, mainly on the humoral immunity.

3   Ozone therapy improved the indices of lipid peroxidation [marker of oxidative cell membrane destruction] without exogenous [externally given] antioxidants.

Tumour PO2 [oxygen pressure] Modification by Ozonetherapy (B. Clavo et al)

Findings support that ozone therapy could be a useful adjuvant in treatment of hypoxic [oxygen deficient] tumours.

Local Ozone Therapy for Delayed Scarring In Cancer Patients (G. Rovira et al)

Local ozone therapy is a useful treatment to: a) accelerate healing wounds in previously irradiated areas b) avoid delays to start chemotherapy and/or radio-therapy in patients with delayed scarring after [cancer] surgery.

Ozone Influence on the Level of Endotoxicosis in General Hyperthermia Condition of Oncologic Patients (G. Boyarinov et al)

Using ozone therapy as a method of oxidative detoxification, it is possible to significantly decrease the degree of endotoxicosis [toxicity released by bacteria as they are destroyed] in oncologic patients...

(Note: related to this abstract is the point of view that oxygen-ozone sauna therapy helps the body to detoxify—which in turn helps the body deal with oxidative stress, and modulate (balance) the immune system. It is thought oxygen-ozone sauna helps the body to detoxify because it assists the body oxidise 'wastes' and toxins. When oxidised, toxins are rendered safe and more easily eliminated from the body.)

Studies carried out up until the present time indicate oxygen-ozone therapy is likely to be a beneficial therapy for individuals with cancer. It has a real part to play as one part of a balanced naturopathic approach to health. However, despite the interest surrounding ozone therapy and cancer, none of these studies indicate that it specifically and directly reverses cancer. Therefore it should always be used in conjunction with other cancer therapies.

Oxygen-ozone therapy is also invaluable for many other illnesses and conditions, from vaginal yeast infections to ulcers and burn wounds. Interestingly ozonated oils, which are quite stable at cool temperatures, allow many of the benefits of oxygen-ozone to be easily transported around. Also of significance is the fact that ozonated oils make an outstanding toothpaste, as its antibacterial and oxygenating effects are very beneficial to the gums.

The International Ozone Association (IOA) has collated many hundreds of studies—and it is worth mentioning one particular small-scale study of ozone's action against MRSA (antibiotic resistant bacteria) skin and bladder infections. Three treatments of oxygen-ozone gas and/or ozonated water proved to be 100% effective at eradicating the infection. (Follow up microbiology reports were carried out between one–twelve weeks after treatment and showed no sign of infection).[21]

Considering conventional medicine is often at a loss as to how to treat such infections, with many individuals who have contracted MRSA having to spend long periods of time in complete isolation—it is a great shame oxygen-ozone treatment is not being more widely utilised.

Cost: In terms of cost, the going rate for ozone steam sauna therapy varies between countries between £35–£45 ($56–$72) a session in the UK compared to £15 (US$24) in Canada. Time in the sauna is usually around ½ hour – forty minutes and most practitioners suggest that you receive the therapy upwards of twice a week, over a significant period of time, if you are dealing with serious illness.

Autohemotherapy is a more expensive option at around £50–£80 ($75–$120) per time in the UK & £31–£42 (US$50–$67) in Canada.

It is possible to purchase your own equipment, (which makes carrying out the therapy twice a week for several months easier and more cost effective). Approx cost of equipment is between £850 ($1360) and £1171 ($1875). See the following link for a list of suppliers:

http://www.dmoz.org/Health/Alternative/Ozone_Therapy

However, if you do purchase your own equipment, it is important you use it correctly and safely. Make sure you are using a safe concentration of ozone (for skin contact applications this is generally less than 30 mcg/ml—mcg/ml meaning micrograms per millilitre) and remember the rule of thumb for ozone therapy: 'stay low & go slow'.

Where to obtain the therapy: Start with a search on a search engine for practitioners offering oxygen ozone sauna therapy. In addition, some of the manufacturers that come up under the URL listed above (such as Ozone Services) will be able to put you in touch with a trained practitioner in your area.

In the UK ozone therapy (in combination with other important non-toxic cancer treatments) can be obtained at:

The Dove Clinic for Integrated Medicine
Hockley Mill Stables
Twyford
Hampshire
S021 1NT

☎: 01962 718000
🖷: 01962 718011

4

Group 2 Therapies –
Non-Clinic Based Cancer Therapies

IN THIS CHAPTER WE WILL look at Group 2 Therapies—therapies that specifically target cancer, which you can carry out in your local area in conjunction with a health professional. We will look in detail at what is involved in carrying out each therapy—again including approximate costs. For some of the therapies we will also look at the underlying theory on which they are based. It was our original intention to look at a number of theories of cancer in a preceding chapter, however because the theories are not essential to understanding about the therapies that are available, we have now moved them to Appendix B: Important Theories Of Cancer (see p.231). Nevertheless, we will refer to particular theories when appropriate and recommend reading them in full at a later time.

Here is a list of the therapies we are going to cover in this chapter. Also included in the table are very approximate cost guidelines of each therapy. Costs are given per month, and where appropriate initial start-up cost as well.

Therapy	Brief description/comments	Cost/month	More details
Natural Anti-Cancer Compounds	With natural compounds it is important that you use them synergistically and in high enough amounts. Decide which natural anti-cancer compounds you are going to take and work up to your target dose slowly.	£15.66 ($25) per day £469.80 ($751) per month.	See p.37
Diet / Food Therapy (Metabolic Typing)	There are many different diets around—however the most important factor is that you follow a diet that is right for your body type. For this reason—we recommend Metabolic Typing. The testing that you will undergo as part of the Metabolic Typing analysis will identify the correct foods & combinations of them that are right for your biochemistry. After the cost of the first months testing procedure the diet (food wise) will probably work out similar to what you currently spend.	£240 ($384) for initial testing and 1st month's follow-up.	See p.55
	Recommended supplements. These are optional in the sense that they complement your particular food type diet.	£150 ($240) per month	
	As you continue on the program you will need to budget for occasional retests and support.	After 1st month, monthly testing and support will work out to about £50 ($80)	
Photodynamic Therapy	Photosensitive compound that accumulates preferentially in cancer cells. Photosensitive compound is activated by light of the correct frequency.	Agent costs approx £166 ($308) per month. Light costs £613 ($1135)	See p.75 & p.146
Burzynski's Aminocare® A10	Marketed primarily as a cancer preventive supplement, Burzynski considers it is also useful as a complementary cancer therapy.	£75 ($120)	See p.77 & p.119

Pancreatic Enzyme supplements	Based on John Beards theory that pancreatic enzymes are needed to unmask trophoblast cells to make them visible to the immune system. Take recommended amounts between meals.	£34 ($55)	See p.68 & p.238
Naessens 714-X Therapy	Cost of 21-day series of injections The 21-day series of injections should be repeated several times with a short break in-between them. Injections can be carried out by yourself as they are very easy and straightforward and go into the lymph system rather than the blood system.	£187 ($300) series of 21 injections.	See p.80
Cantron	A formulation specially designed to cause cancer cells to die off. Cantron is also the worlds most powerful antioxidant.	£26 ($47)	See p.90
B-17/Amygdalin	B-17 / Amygdalin / Laetrile Intravenous infusion of Laetrile is the best choice if you can locate a practitioner who performs it. Second best are laetrile tablets, and your last choice (though not really recommended), raw apricot kernels. B-17, taken orally, should always be taken on an empty stomach.	UK cost approx £90 each. US cost approx $100 each. £89 ($142) for laetrile tablets (500mg x 3 a day) £10 ($16) for apricot kernels	See p.99 & p.238
Hydrazine Sulphate	Based on a breaking the 'sick' relationship between a cancer patients liver and their cancer.	£27.50 ($44)	See p.102

Table 4: Group 2 Therapies—Therapies That Can Be Carried Out Locally

We will now take a look in more detail at each of the therapies listed in the above table.

Natural Anti-Cancer Compounds Discussed By John Boik

John Boik is a cancer researcher who has recently published a groundbreaking study on natural compounds and their potential use as a cancer therapy. His work entitled 'Natural Compounds in Cancer Therapy' (Oregon Medical Press, 2001) is particularly important for several reasons. In particular Boik:

- Identifies and clarifies ways in which natural compounds are able to exert a therapeutic influence on cancer cells.

- Identifies that to achieve a therapeutic effect, natural compounds need to be used synergistically (i.e. combinations of multiple compounds used together at the same time). Boik suggests combinations of fifteen or more natural compounds.

- Calculates, for the first time, the approximate oral intake required for each of thirty-six different natural compounds to become therapeutically active against cancer cells. (Calculations are approximate as they are based on present research, and may therefore be subject to revision in the future.)

For many important compounds, Boik has synthesised the results of different studies and attempted to resolve inconsistencies between them. In his latest book, Boik references over four thousand studies.

In this section we will examine points 1–3 above in more detail. (For detailed information about point 4—please see Boik's book). Let us begin with what Boik calls the 'seven clusters of procancer events'. These are the different events that promote the development of cancer in the first place. You will see in the table below, along with each procancer event, we have also listed its corresponding 'antidote' (i.e. remedy). Having a sense of these 'clusters of procancer events' will help you understand more, the type of factors that contribute to the development of cancer, as well as illuminate therapeutic avenues worth pursuing. Also, in the interview with Boik later in this section, we will use this table as the framework for our discussion.

As will become clearer as we progress through this section, each of the above 'clusters of procancer events' is an area that can be addressed therapeutically with the use of natural compounds. For example, some natural compounds help with DNA stability by reducing oxidative stress (i.e. free radical stress—free

Procancer Events	Inhibition Strategy
Genetic instability (lack of DNA stability) leads to increased cellular mutations and an increased ability of cells to adapt to immune attacks mounted by the body & by cancer therapies.	Reduce genetic instability by reducing oxidative stress (i.e. reducing excess of free radicals) at cancer sites and within the body generally.
Abnormal gene (sections of the cellular DNA) expression leading to the production of proteins that stimulate cancer cell growth & proliferation.	Improve the integrity of the cell components that read DNA and generate proteins, with the aim of reducing the generation of proteins that stimulate cancer growth & proliferation.
Abnormal signalling and communication between the outside of a cell and its inner workings. This abnormal signalling leads to cancer cells being instructed to proliferate.	Aim to reduce the intensity & frequency of signalling, as it is generally excessive in cancerous cells.
Abnormal cell-to-cell communication, that leads to aberrant cell behaviour.	Encourage cellular communication so cells act as part of a community rather than acting independently.
Excessive stimulation of angiogenesis (growth of new blood vessels) leading to better oxygen and nutrient delivery to cancer cells.	Provide factors that can limit the process of angiogenesis to a more normal level.
Invasion and metastasis (spreading) of cancer cells through the body leading to expansion and proliferation of tumours.	Limiting invasion by inhibiting the release of enzymes from cancer cells that dissolve surrounding tissue. Metastasis can be targeted in a number of ways including increasing the ability of the immune system to identify and target rogue cells, as well as by improving the health of blood vessels.
Cellular evasion of the immune system leading to unchecked growth and proliferation of cancer cells.	A duel strategy is proposed of increasing immune system response, while at the same time reducing cancer cells ability to remain invisible.

Table 5: Procancer Events & Their Possible 'Antidotes'[22]

radicals are atoms, or groups of atoms, possessing an unpaired electron and hence are very reactive), some compounds help with cell-to-cell communication and others help by reducing the growth of new blood vessels etc.

Boik has focused on thirty-six promising natural compounds, and for each compound (with reference to studies that have been carried out) establishes what anti-cancer actions it possesses and how it can help therapeutically (i.e. how it fits into the table above). We can note that many of the thirty-six compounds Boik investigates are able to exert a whole spectrum of anti-cancer activity and are therefore able to address several of the clusters listed in the table at the same time. This is to be welcomed because the general principle we are working to is that it is best to 'attack' cancer on many fronts at once. Boik notes this is how 'Nature' works herself, and also that it is important to build 'redundancy' into any therapy, so that if one compound fails to act against its 'target', others are automatically available to fulfil the same role.

Let us now examine the concept of synergism because it is so central to Boik's approach. Synergism refers to the use of multiple compounds, at the same time. Synergism is a concept long utilised by traditional herbalism and herbal formulas generally contain several different ingredients. Traditionally, rather than use single ingredient formulas, herbalists have preferred formulas made up of multiple ingredients in specific proportions to each other. Regarding the value of synergism, it turns out that herbalists have been on to a good thing for a long time. To explain exactly why this is, we need to look at the limitations of using a single natural compound rather than combinations of compounds to achieve a therapeutic effect.

The main problem with using a single natural compound for treatment is that if the compound is to remain non-toxic, then it is difficult to reach blood concentrations necessary for therapeutic effect to occur. Of course, one of the main reasons for using natural compounds instead of pharmaceutical cancer drugs is to avoid issues of toxicity—so there is no point in giving natural compounds at levels that cause toxicity and damage to the body. For this reason the safe level of ingestion of any particular compound, limits the blood concentration obtainable. Secondly, the oral route of administration (rather than the intravenous route) tends to limit the concentration of a compound that can build up in the blood stream. This can be due to inefficiencies in the assimilation of the compound, or because a primary compound is metabolised by the liver into secondary compounds—thereby limiting the level of the first.

However when natural compounds are utilised synergistically (i.e. together) it is as though a little magic happens—the end result being that we are able to overcome the blood concentration problems associated with using a single natural compound. Looking at it mathematically, the theory of synergism states that $1 + 1 + 1 = 6$ or 8 or 10—but not the usual mathematical 3. That is: the whole is greater than the sum of its parts. This is the principle we can use to overcome the gap that usually exists between the maximum blood concentration obtainable with non-toxic use of a compound, and the level needed for therapeutic effect. And, in line with this principle, the more compounds we use the greater the synergistic effect will become.

Synergism is a concept that is relatively new and uncharted in the field of modern science. The main reason being that it isn't easy to study, because modern science is founded upon experiments where all the variables except one are kept completely constant, and the effect noted of varying this single experimental variable. How is science to deal with ten, fifteen or twenty experimental variables working together? To this end, Boik has made a start in this study, and one particular experiment he has conducted shows the principle of synergism working well.

We will simplify the terminology of the experiment to make it easier to communicate. Boik took twelve natural compounds and first measured the concentration of each needed to achieve a therapeutic effect. Totalled up, the 'amount' of compounds used came to eighteen units. Boik then mixed the compounds together and re-measured the concentration needed for the same 'therapeutic effect' to occur. Boik found that when used together their power was magnified 4½ times—and so needed the equivalent of only four units of the compounds (when added together) to achieve the same effect.

It is this synergistic effect that makes it possible to use natural compounds therapeutically—without it they would most likely be too weak acting. It also means it is essential to build up a therapeutic program consisting of enough elements. As mentioned, Boik considers around fifteen to eighteen is a reasonable number when taking into account all the factors of synergism, addressing the seven clusters of procancer events listed in the table and building in redundancy.

Also, Boik suggests using a number of compounds that are 'direct acting', some that are 'indirect acting' and some that are 'immune system stimulants'. The term 'Immune system stimulants' is self-explanatory—but 'direct acting' refers to compounds that directly act against cancer cells (e.g. reduce excessive internal cellular signals that are instructing a cancer cell to grow and divide). 'Indirect acting' refers to compounds that exert their action via the environment they create around cancer cells (e.g. compounds that can reduce oxidative stress in the body and hence improve DNA stability).

Boik's whole approach is based around 'coaxing' cancer cells back into the 'fold'. His view is that research over the last decade has identified ways in which cancer cells are different from normal healthy cells—and that an ideal approach for cancer therapy is to attempt to help cancer cells 'become more normal'—to return to the fold, so to speak. Cancer cells have left the 'community of cells' and struck out on their own. Boik is therefore suggesting that, rather than try to directly kill cancer cells, we should instead provide a range of natural factors to

Choice	Compound	Research indicated range
Direct Acting Compounds that act directly upon cancer cells		
2 of 4	Apigenin – plant flavonoid	0.1 – 0.6 g per day
	Luteolin – plant flavonoid	0.17 – 1.8 g per day
	Genistein – isoflavonoid (high in soy)	0.1 – 1.1 g per day
	Quercetin – plant flavonoid	0.25 – 1.8 g per day
1 of 2	Arctigenin – active compound burdock seed	0.65 g per day
	Arctium seed – burdock seed	12 g per day
1 of 2	Boswellic acid – active comp. Frankincense	1.8 g per day
	Asiatic acid (from Centella) – herb gotu kola	1.7 g per day
1 of 1	CAPE – active compound bee propolis	3 – 15 g per day
1 of 1	Curcumin – active ingredient in tumeric	1.5 – 1.8 g per day
1 of 1	Emodin – active ingredient of some herbs	0.16 – 0.81 g per day
1 of 1	EPA/DHA – omega-3 fatty acids from fish oil	6 – 21 g per day
0 of 1	Garlic (or 4mg allicin potential for each gram)	6 – 15 g per day
1 of 3	Limonene – from fragrant essential oils	7.3 – 14 g per day
	Perillyl alcohol - from fragrant essential oils	1.3 – 9 g per day
	Geraniol – from fragrant essential oils	0.27 – 5.7 g per day
1 of 1	Parthenolide – active compound herb feverfew	17 mg per day
1 of 1	Resveratrol – compound in wine & grapes	68 – 410 mg per day
1 of 1	Selenium – trace element	250 – 1100 µg per day
1 of 1	Vitamin A emulsified as retinyl esters	50000 – 600000 i.u/day
1 of 1	Vitamin D3 in form of 1,25-D3	0.75 – 2.5 µg per day
1 of 2	Vitamin E – primary antioxidant	440 – 1700 i.u per day
	Vitamin E succinate – more useful form	440 – 1700 i.u per day
Indirect-Acting Compounds (action by influencing the cancer cells environment)		
1 of 2	Anthocyanidins – red-blue pigments	0.12 – 1.8 g per day
	Proanthocyanidins – grape seed bioflavonoid	0.49 – 1.8 g per day
1 of 2	Ruscogenins from butcher's broom	100 – 130 mg per day
	Aesin extract from horse chestnut	150 mg per day
0 of 1	Vitamin C – primary antioxidant	1 – 2 g per day
Immune Stimulants (compounds that enhance the immune system)		
1 of 1	Bromelain or enzyme mix	1 – 4 g per day
1 of 1	Astragalus membranaceus – 7% polysaccharide	Include in PSP/PSK amt
1 of 2	Siberian ginseng - 7% polysaccharides	Include in PSP/PSK amt
	Panax ginseng – active ingredient ginsenoside	110-340mg ginsenoside
1 of 3	PSP/PSK (dose < 3g crude extract)	2–9g of polysaccharides /day. Polysacch. approx 7% of raw product
	Ganoderma – (dose < 1.9g crude extract)	
	Shiitake – immunostimulating mushroom	
1 of 1	Melatonin – sleep inducing hormone	3 – 20 mg per day
0 of 1	Glutamine – amino acid	8 – 30 g per day
Compounds For Which The Required Dose Is Relatively Uncertain		
0 of 3	EGCG – active compound in green tea extract	0.46 – 0.55 g per day
	Flaxseed – for lignans & alpha-linolenic acid	30–60g/day (ground up)
	Hypericin – active comp. St John's Wort	5.6 – 11 mg per day

Table 6: Compounds Boik Discusses Including Preliminary Research Indicated Intake[23]

enable them to either die a natural death (as aberrant cells are programmed to do), or to rejoin the community of cells and play a valuable role.

Before we examine the list of Boik's suggested natural compounds, we should note that the dosages listed are preliminary estimates. This is the first time such detailed calculations have been made and it may be that some of the dosage guidelines will change with time (Boik lists updates on his website). In the table below, you will find substances listed in groups of similar acting compounds (i.e. potentially redundant compounds). For each of these groups of similar acting compounds, a recommendation is made of how many might reasonably be added to a therapeutic protocol.

You will notice that the 'Research Indicated Range' for each compound is significantly higher than would normally be recommended—and this is representative of the work Boik has carried out in determining intakes that are necessary to exert a therapeutic effect against cancer cells (when used synergistically). You may be wondering why the dosages listed in the table are so high, when previously we have described that synergism, due to its magnification effect, is able to reduce the dose of each individual compound required. However, the dosages listed are in fact far lower than that indicated if they were to be used alone and *not* synergistically (around a fifteen fold reduction for each compound).

You will also note the arrangement of compounds into groups—and if you select one item out of every group (where at least one item is recommended), you will find the total comes to twenty-two items. These twenty-two items will help with the design of a therapeutic program, which address all the seven levels of procancer events listed in Table 5: Procancer Events & Their Possible 'Antidotes' (see p.35).

Before we look in more detail at using these natural compound recommendations, we would like to reference the point mentioned at the beginning of this section regarding Boik's synthesis of various studies—specifically studies on vitamin C as an anti-cancer agent. Over recent decades there has been controversy about the value of vitamin C as a cancer therapy. After considering all the arguments, Boik considers a dose of between one to two grams a day appropriate and that it is best used as part of a comprehensive program rather than as a single compound therapy. You will find an outline of the arguments in favour of using mega-doses of vitamin C as a cancer therapy in Appendix A: Additional Well Known Cancer Therapies.

How to use the recommendations

Our recommendation is that you should put Boik's recommendations into practice in conjunction with your physician and/or health professional. To find a physician/health professional in your area who is open to this kind of approach, please see the 'Find Practitioner' section of www.ompress.com (Boik's website) or see Appendix C: Useful Contacts & Resources for other physician listings.

There are a few compounds listed in the table that need special mention. This is because they may produce allergic reactions or because an individual needs vigilant monitoring when taking such a large dose. The compounds this applies to are CAPE (an extract of bee propolis), selenium, vitamin A and enzymes. Enzymes in particular should not be taken within twenty-four hours of surgery, used by individuals on anticoagulants or with an increased heart rate.[24] Also we should note that melatonin is best taken before going to bed, while the other compounds are best taken in measured portions three or four times a day. An overall schedule of fifteen days on and then a five-day rest period is suggested. Pregnant women or women who are breast-feeding should, of course, use all of the mentioned compounds with extreme care.

In addition, individuals dealing with oestrogen-dependant tumours are advised to avoid genistein (most usually a soya bean derivative)—as there is a chance it might promote tumour growth. Other estrogenic compounds in the list such as panax ginseng, flaxseed and resveratrol are considered to exert a much milder estrogenic effect, but you may still do best avoiding them if you have an oestrogen dependant tumour.[25,26]

The recommended daily intake refers to the actual active compound named in the table. In most cases these are not available as 100% pure formulations—rather they are available in the form of standardised extracts. For instance curcumin is commonly available as an 80–90% standardised extract, whereas emodin is only available as a 10% standardised extract. This needs to be borne in mind when calculating how many capsules or tablets of a particular substance to take a day.

Standardised extracts have certain advantages over pure formulations in that they retain much of the chemical complexity of their original source. Even if an extract is standardised to 90%, the other 10% is likely to contain other beneficial and supportive compounds. In contrast, a 100% pure formulation will not contain any additional compounds. Also, some supplements may contain a couple of the suggested compounds. For instance an emodin standardised extract (10%) may also contain resveratrol at 20%. Thus you may need to do a few calculations to obtain the substances at appropriate levels.

More about obtaining the compounds.

Most of the compounds can be obtained from internet suppliers. It is just a case of entering the compound name in a search engine and checking out what different suppliers have to offer. You can find a list of suppliers on Boik's website at: www.ompress.com/main-products.htm as well as some supplemental information in Appendix C: Useful Contacts & Resources (p.249). We can note that all of the above compounds are reasonably easy to obtain, except for standardised apigenin and standardised CAPE. We recommend you obtain a copy of Boik's book and discuss the contents with your health professional. It is very readable and contains far more detail than we are able to cover here.

Costs: The cost of following such a program is quite difficult to ascertain—because each person is likely to pick out different substances. However, we have done some calculations and a reasonable selection works out to approximately £15.66 ($25.06) per day. Please see Appendix D: Natural Compounds Against Cancer Costings (p.253) for more about compound costings and suppliers.

Interview with John Boik (Natural Compounds & Cancer)

SK: Thank you John for agreeing to give this interview. In terms of a general structure, I am thinking we can use your seven clusters of procancer events—and also their possible 'antidotes'. As we work our way through these, I am sure we can cover other related points.

John Boik: Fine, but if I may, I would like to make a couple of general comments first.

The field of cancer research has changed. In fact it has been changing dramatically over the last five to ten years. Not so long ago, the main focus was on cytotoxic [cell killing] chemotherapy. That's what everybody was doing—that's what everyone was studying. Now, by and large, the focus has shifted to targeting the molecular events occurring within a cancer cell that distinguish it from a normal one—the kind of things I talk about in my book.

I don't mean to say that cytotoxic chemotherapy is useless. On the contrary, there are certain cancers that it works wonders on—but I think that in the near future we will be coming up with far more beneficial approaches. These may incorporate some cytotoxic [cell killing] chemotherapy, but are likely to contain many other additional elements as well. Natural plant compounds could be a part too—it's possible that some could work really well with chemotherapy or with the other new drugs under development, and make them more effective.

SK: You mean that instead of studying and researching how to kill cancer cells using chemotherapy compounds, research has shifted, to study in more depth the actual workings of a cancer cell to find out how it varies from a normal cell—and how these differences can be addressed therapeutically?

JB: Yes—exactly. For the last decade or more, researchers have been looking at the million-dollar question of 'what makes a cancer cell different from a normal cell?'

And as basic science has been finding answers to this question, new targets for cancer therapy have arisen. So now there's a whole new generation of drugs coming out that promise to be far less toxic to an individual and far more specific to cancer cells.

People are talking about the need for using more than one drug at a time. I've heard the word 'synergism' tossed around quite a bit—and I would say that synergism is the new frontier in cancer research. That is, using mixtures of agents to try to attack the cancer cell on many different levels at once. This is exactly what I discuss in my book—the possibility of using mixtures of natural, relatively mild-acting compounds that can target cancer cells, but leave normal cells unharmed.

SK: I found the evidence you presented on synergism very compelling. I understand that the concept of synergism comes from traditional herbalism—where a remedy is made up from a number of different natural compounds. In fact there are often quite intense debates over the best makeup of a particular remedy in terms of its constituents and proportions.

That is why I found your experiment into synergism described in the book so interesting. If I am correct, you took twelve compounds and determined the concentration at which they individually became active against cancer cells in the test tube—and then found the active concentration needed for a mixture containing all twelve compounds together. The mixture was effective at a concentration about four times lower than what would be expected if the effects of each compound were only additive—its power was magnified about four times over that expected. As I said, I found this very interesting—it is the first experiment I have read of, where the principle of synergism has been investigated.

JB: Yes, synergism is the effect when you add one plus one together and get six or seven or ten or something greater than two. Basically the whole is greater that the sum of its parts—that's what synergism is all about.

   I'm trying to bring the study of synergism into the world of natural medicine, as well as encourage it within conventional science. Although the concept is old, it has not received its fair share of research; in cancer medicine the term synergism is still a frontier buzzword. Especially with regard to mixtures of more than two agents, research is just getting off the ground.

SK: I am thinking that science has an immediate problem with synergism because there are too many factors to account for in the experiment. The foundation of modern day science is that all variables except one are kept constant. This allows us to see the effect upon outcome of this single variable. Any more than one variable becomes a real headache.

JB: Yes, that's exactly the problem. There actually have been quite a number of synergism studies done in the test tube on two drugs, and even some on two natural compounds, for example vitamins A and D3. But when you're talking about mixing more than two or three compounds together— basically it's uncharted territory. This is interesting because humans evolved using herbal mixtures that probably contained dozens or even hundreds of active compounds. So for all our ability to put a person on the moon—we still barely understand how four compounds might interact to produce a biological effect.

SK: Well—that feels like a good outline of synergy for us to work with. I would like to suggest that we begin with the first item listed in your table of procancer events—genetic instability. Can you say a bit about this and how it can be targeted therapeutically.

JB: Our DNA holds the pattern for each cell's behaviour and function. For the most part, the makeup and expression of a cell's DNA is held relatively stable—it doesn't change that much. That's a good thing, because you don't want mutations in DNA structure that lead to cancer, nor do you want changes in DNA expression that lead to inappropriate function. For example, you don't want your muscle cells acting like liver or kidney cells.

   But the DNA within cancer cells tends to be particularly pliable—and that's because the watchdogs, (the genes that make sure that the DNA is kept stable), are often themselves mutated. This allows greater flexibility in the genetic code of cancer cells.

   In turn, this gives them the wonderful ability, from their standpoint, to quickly adapt—and as conditions change, they can change as well. Even a small tumour contains millions of cancer cells, and due to genetic alterations not every one of these cells will be the same. If you expose the tumour to a drug it is likely that one or more of its cells are going to be naturally immune. Maybe they don't have the receptor, or the enzyme, or the protein the drug works on. So even though the drug might kill the vast majority of cells in the tumour—some of the cells are likely to survive. These will repopulate, resulting in a new drug-resistant tumour.

Similarly, some drugs or conditions (such as oxidative stress) that damage DNA can themselves lead to increased mutation rates, thereby compounding the problem.

SK: It's almost as if from an evolutionary, adaptive viewpoint, cancer cells are more efficient?

JB: It is like instant evolution—near instant evolution. That is one of the primary reasons why cancer is so difficult to stop. You don't have a fixed target—rather the target is always changing.

SK: So how can natural compounds influence DNA stability? How do they help?

JB: As an example, oxidative stress is one of the elements that can produce an environment that favours genetic pliability. At least in theory, reducing oxidative stress at a tumour site may reduce the forces pushing the genetic evolution along.

Although this is still theoretical, it seems reasonable based on pre-clinical evidence. If correct, then use of natural antioxidant or anti-inflammatory compounds, of which there are many, could reduce the ability of a cancer cell to adapt.

I was having dinner with a friend the other night, and he had spent a fair amount of time in Thailand. He said the Thai people were really wonderful and they had a way about them in that they didn't attack problems directly. Rather, they skilfully wooed a solution out of any given problem. He said they have a very soft but effective approach.

For example, when they wanted to slaughter a wild pig, they didn't run after it to chase it down—rather what they did was to put out a little bait on a string- and by pulling the string at the right moments, encourage the pig to come to where they wanted it. The whole job would be done with hardly any 'squealing'. Instead of just being the target, the pig became part of the process.

Maybe it is a useful concept for cancer—maybe the best way to treat cancer is to coax it out of its aggressive behaviour.

SK: To try to gently pull it or nudge it back into the fold?

JB: Exactly—and that takes us into another one of the events that I have listed in the book: cell-to-cell communication. One of the first things that happen when a cell becomes neoplastic [i.e. starts growing abnormally] is that it loses touch with its neighbours. All cells have proteins on their surface that act as hands to feel and communicate with their environment. As a cancer cell loses communication with healthy cells, it takes on more and more aggressive behaviour. In fact, altering nothing else in cancer cells but the genes to encourage cell-to-cell communication can lead to loss of aggressive qualities. Cancer cells will behave more like normal cells if you can get them to talk with their neighbours.

SK: I was really struck by your description of the breakdown of communication between cancer cells and their neighbours. Cancer is often described as 'the' disease of our civilization—and on one level cancer cells do exhibit the very spirit of our times—i.e. the breakdown of community. Not that I wish to infer in any way that someone's personality who contracts cancer is in any way anti-community or anti-communication… but to a certain extent cancer is like a mirroring of the spirit of the age.

JB: In many ways a cancer cell is like a damaged and troubled youth who has divorced himself or herself from the community—the cell becomes a rebel and selfish—just looking out for its own best interests. Whether we are talking about a community of cells or a community of human beings, communities have to work together—and communities help to keep their members functioning in a way that's healthy for the whole.

SK: Can some natural compounds help encourage cell-to-cell communication?

JB: Yes, there are several. Cell-to-cell communication is a result of various proteins and enzymes at work—and a number of natural compounds have been shown to effect those proteins and enzymes in such a way to encourage cell-to-cell communication.

SK: What you described about 'do not die' signals coming from cell-to-cell contact was fascinating. You explain that most cells need to receive 'do not die' signals from adjacent cells to stay alive; these balance out the ever present 'do die' signals built into each cell. Therefore, when the cancer cell breaks away to go it alone it has to manufacture its own 'do not die' signals if it to survive.

JB: Yes, quite right. Most cells die when taken away from their neighbours because they do not receive enough 'do not die' signals. There's always a precarious balance of 'do die' and 'do not die' signals occurring in a cell.

But cancer cells mutate in such a way that they are able to generate their own 'do not die' signals. Whether that's through the production of growth factors or some other method, they find a way to tell themselves not to die. Therefore they tend to live a longer life, and by doing so have greater opportunity for producing offspring.

By the way, most cancer cells don't actually grow much faster than normal cells. There is a common misconception that cancer cells proliferate far more quickly than other cells of the body. Actually, the cells of most cancers proliferate no faster than those of other fast-growing normal tissues, such as the bone marrow, hair follicles, or intestinal lining. The problem is more that they live too long and thus have many more chances to produce offspring. Most current chemotherapy drugs target fast-growing cells; hence they induce side effects in the other fast-growing tissues [e.g. chemotherapy causing hair to fall out].

SK: OK... The next item on the table is the abnormal expression of genes. Maybe you could explain what 'expression of a gene means'?

JB: Gene expression is really nothing more than sections of the DNA being used as a template to produce a protein. That's all. The DNA contains a large number of genes, and most genes, when expressed, produce a protein. Proteins are the workhorses of a cell. If something needs to be done such as movement, proliferation or almost any other event, then proteins make it happen. Protein turnover in a cell can be rapid, so new proteins are usually needed for new actions.

SK: Particular proteins carry out specific functions?

JB: Yes, each protein carries out a certain function—proteins are responsible for thousands of different functions within a cell.

One of the things that help turn on and off a gene to make a protein is a number of little proteins called transcription factors—and some natural compounds can affect transcription factor function. In fact, natural compounds can affect nearly every part of the machinery of gene expression and thus can affect protein production.

So if a mutated cell is producing an abnormal protein or abnormal amounts of a protein—and let's say it is a protein that is giving the cell survival signals (i.e. 'do not die' signals), it may be possible to use natural compounds to interrupt the process and reduce the signals.

SK: And signal transduction (the next item in the table of procancer events)—that's the communication of signals from the outside of the cell to the nucleus in the centre of the cell.

JB: Yes, signals are passed along in a cell by proteins, much the same way that runners pass along a baton in a relay race. The goal in the case of the cell is often some kind of event within the nucleus. Whether it's production of a protein from the DNA, or some other activity, the signal starts at one place in the cell and is carried to another.

An example is the survival signals we already talked about [the 'do not dies signals']. Commonly, these signals are initiated by growth factors that touch receptors on the outside of the cell. The chemical signal is carried, much like the baton, to the centre of the cell. Along the way, the signal has to pass through many hands, and each of these is a target for therapy. There are several natural compounds that can affect the enzymes or other proteins that make up the relay hands.

SK: I am wondering about effects on healthy cells of introducing these natural compounds. Are signal transduction, gene expression, or cell-to-cell communication in healthy cells going to be negatively affected by these compounds?

JB: That's a good question. Ideally of course, we want to develop therapies that are specific to cancer cells so that normal ones are not harmed. I'll use signal transduction as an example here.

Most normal cells don't replicate all that often, and not unless they're instructed to do so by their environment. When conditions are right and replication is needed, proliferation signals have to go through the whole relay cascade that we described earlier.

One thing that makes a cancer cell different is that it is flooded with signals. In large part this is because it can produce its own growth factors—the process of self-stimulation. It's flooded in messages saying 'live, live, live', and 'produce, produce, produce'. Another difference is that cancer cells tend to over-use a small number of pathways in the signalling chain. If we relate it to the runners race—one particular lane will be used heavily and have lots of traffic on it.

So if we give compounds that slow the signalling down, particularly over the heavily used pathways, a cancer cell would be severely affected whereas normal cells would not be harmed.

SK: That's a helpful analogy John—so out of the seven procancer cluster events, we have now discussed four of them. I would say the ones we have discussed are the more technical ones. I'm thinking that the three left (angiogenesis, metastasis and immune evasion) are, in a sense, much easier to relate to. Let's talk about angiogenesis first.

JB: Yes, the remaining events are more what we might call 'big-picture' events. For instance I think most people will understand metastasis as the spread of tumour cells from one place in the body to another.

Let's look at angiogenesis. It is a hot topic in cancer research—a very hot topic. Angiogenesis is the growth of new blood vessels, a process that is critical for a tumour to grow. To get much bigger than a millimetre in diameter, a tumour needs to attract blood vessels that supply it with nutrients and oxygen. If those blood vessels don't grow then a tumour doesn't grow. So cancer cells have figured out a way to produce the specific growth factors and other compounds that induce capillaries to grow towards them.

SK: Shark cartilage has been the agent promoted in the 'alternative' field for several years as an agent than can reduce angiogenesis. There are several trials being conducted into its efficacy at the present time and the results are due in a couple of years. Some mainstream critics have been very hostile to the use of shark cartilage to target angiogenesis—what is happening in the research world?

JB: I would say very few angiogenesis researchers are concerned whether or not shark cartilage works—it has very little bearing on the field as a whole. Most researchers are concerned with endostatins [naturally occurring antiangiogenic proteins] and other compounds that have well-docu-mented effects on angiogenesis. So the reaction to shark cartilage hasn't affected research on angiogenesis.

Now, I would like to say that angiogenesis provides a good example of why a multi-tiered therapeutic approach is important. In the research studies using antiangiogenic drugs, some truly remarkable results have been shown in animals—and I mean truly remarkable. They've shown that tumours in mice will completely regress and stay away as long as the drug is given.

But these drugs don't seem to work so well in humans. The early trials with antiangiogenic compounds have actually been quite disappointing. One reason for this is that human tumours tend to be well established and slower growing than the experimental animal tumours, so they are not so dependent on development of new blood supplies. And even if the growth of new vessels were prevented, the ones that are already established will continue to feed the tumour and keep it alive.

So the animal results were more profound than the human results. The lesson is, on their own, antiangiogenic drugs should not be expected to stop an established human tumour, and this brings us back to the multi-tiered approach.

SK: How do you see a multi-tiered approach best employed for a person with cancer?

JB: It seems to me, every major part of tumour development should be simultaneously targeted. Angiogenesis could be targeted, but only along with other aspects of cancer biology, like cell-to-cell communication and the signal transduction pathways we have discussed. One could address all seven of the areas that I list in the book, as appropriate for a given type of cancer.

SK: I understand that angiogenesis is a natural process the body uses during wound healing. What I found so illuminating is the way that cancer cells co-opt or mimic everyday processes of the various normal cell types. It's as if cancer cells are able to use any normal function that a cell can exhibit to serve their own end.

JB: That's right. In some senses, cancer cells are truly 'remarkable'. There is probably nothing that a cancer cell does that is not natural to at least some normal cell in the body. For example, cancer cells invade local tissues, but so do blood vessel cells during wound healing…

SK: Related to this, I want to ask you a question. Every time I read about cancer cells, I get the impression they are very sophisticated, and that they can manage sophisticated tasks. And yet, it is generally said they are a genetic mistake. How can these two be reconciled?

JB: From a bird's eye view they appear to be quite sophisticated—amazingly intelligent—as if they have volition. But the biological reality is different. They simply have a pliable genetic code—so each is a little different—and the 'fit' ones survive. As the tumour population encounters new stresses, 'fit' cells survive and prosper and in this way nearly any obstacle is overcome. As an aside, simple survival-of-the-fittest algorithms can be used in computers to solve incredibly complex mathematical problems. The process of survival-of-the-fittest holds tremendous power.

SK: But it seems that cancer cells in different people use the same basic strategies for avoiding the immune system and taking over the body.

JB: It is true to a degree. There are common strategies because through the principle of survival-of-the-fittest, these are the ones that work best.

Large mutations (i.e. ones that would drastically alter a cell's protein makeup and function) are usually rewarded with death. And even if a drastically mutated cell lived, it would be easier for the immune system to recognize it as foreign.

Thus, there tend to be 'workable' mutations commonly found, although these occur in large number. It is like Occam's Razor—all things being equal, the simplest mutations that confers survival will be the ones that work best. And the ones that work best will be the ones passed on to future generations.

So the repertoire of what a cancer cell can do is probably limited to some degree. They can crawl like an immune cell, invade like a blood vessel cell... but they can't jump like a frog...

SK: OK—let's apply what we are talking about to the last two procancer events—metastasis and immune evasion.

JB: Metastasis is the spread of a cancer from one part of the body to another, and actually, it's what kills people. It is rare that a primary tumour kills, except for limited types of cancer. With most cancers, for example with breast cancer, its metastasis to the bone or brain or other areas that causes the most damage. So stopping metastasis is critical if we are to stop cancer—and there's a whole cascade of events that must successfully take place for metastasis to occur. It's not an easy process at all and as a matter of fact there can be literally millions of cancer cells floating in the blood stream of a person with a tumour—but only a very small percentage of these actually take root some place else. With so many things to go wrong, further increasing the challenges to the travelling cells can reduce the rate of metastasis even further.

Of course if a person has an advanced disease that's already metastasised then perhaps trying to stop further metastasis is not a priority—at that point the concern may be to stop the growth of the metastatic tumour. But certainly in early stages stopping metastasis is critical.

SK: How would natural compounds help with preventing metastasis?

JB: There's dozens of ways that you could try to interfere with the metastatic cascade. Taking one example—tumour cells tend to stop in the blood-stream at places where blood vessels are damaged. In animal studies, metastasis tends to be greater in bruised tissues than normal ones. So if you can use a natural compound to strengthen the blood vessels or help repair their damage—then it would stand to reason that the risk of metastasis would be reduced in those areas. The clinical implications of this approach still need to be thoroughly investigated, but it is reasonable to think it could be useful.

SK: And immune evasion—it's surprising cancer cells can camouflage themselves so well…

JB: Yes, yet another amazing ability of cancer cells is that they can hide from the immune system. It is expected of course, based on observation. If the immune system was successful then you wouldn't have cancers progressing in the first place—they would have been destroyed or kept in check.

Quite likely the immune system does attack a new tumour, but those cells that cannot hide are quickly killed and the ones that can hide repopulate the tumour. There are many ways cancer cells can hide, for example they can shed their surface antigens [outside identification markers] so they become unnoticeable. Or they can produce extra antigens and shed so many that nearby immune cells become distracted—a sort of decoy technique. Yet another method is to secrete immunosuppressive compounds in their local area to make immune cells less effective.

Again we come back to the idea that we can use natural compounds to make it harder for cancer cells to hide. Then the immune system will do a better job at finding and destroying them.

SK: In your book, you discuss enzymes in some depth. Is it in relation to targeting cancer cell's ability to evade the immune system you see them as being useful?

JB: I spoke of bromelain and some other compounds. Bromelain is an ingredient of pineapple and there's some pre-clinical work suggesting that it can have a regulatory effect on the immune system. It tends to assist weak cellular responses and subdue excessive ones. And there are other ways to affect the immune system too. For example I've mentioned that cancer cells can release immunosuppressive compounds. Some of these tend to be compounds that also increase inflammation, and in this regard it might be possible to use anti-inflammatory compounds. Fish oil and curcumin are examples.

The trick of course is to take all of this information, put it together, and fit it appropriately to a person needing treatment—that's where there are still a lot of question marks. But it seems to me that the logic behind this approach is sound—and if we keep working one day we will find the way to make it effective.

SK: So, summarizing what we have spoken about so far—the essence is, by using a multi-tiered approach we are really attacking the enemy on all fronts.

JB: Yes, it is that, and more. Terrorism, like cancer, is on the mind of many people these days. How do you fight terrorists? It seems to me the best way is to improve the health of the community that they live in, use police tactics to remove the worst offenders, and encourage the others to rejoin society. What will not work, I believe, is indiscriminate action—poisoning and stressing the community as a whole, trying to break the terrorist roots. With regards to cancer, such an approach (i.e. cytotoxic chemotherapy) has failed and our lessons of the last few decades have been humbling. Crude, forceful approaches have not been successful except in limited instances. To be highly successful, we must understand why a cancer cell is produced, how it lives, how it interacts with its neighbours, how it changes over time, and what makes it different from healthy cells. Then we can begin to find eloquent treatments that harm the cancer and spare the patient. I believe that mixtures of natural compounds can play a role here. They promise to synergistically inhibit cancer by attacking from many angles at once, improve the health of normal tissues, and all the while be non-toxic to the patient. I might add that they could be affordable and available on a worldwide scale.

SK: Some mainstream medical professionals will have a resistance to this soft power approach—they argue that cancer is too strong an adversary and you've got to get in there and kill it stone dead. Could a softer approach really be successful?

JB: Especially in America we tend to have that John Wayne 'get out your six guns and go in shooting' type of attitude. And while it's true that cancer is a very difficult disease, I don't believe that this is necessarily the best approach. Developing a successful softer approach will not be easy, it will take a lot of hard work, but in the end I believe it will be the most successful. To this I might add that cancer need not be viewed as a life-or-death disease. Like diabetes, it may well be possible to live with the disease for a full lifetime if it can be kept in check. In fact this occurs already with many prostate cancer patients, for example. Most elderly men who die of non-cancerous diseases show evidence of prostate cancer. They have it but it does not grow fast enough to give them problems. The important question that researchers now face is how to use non-toxic compounds to keep cancer from spreading and growing.

SK: Let's discuss about the proliferation of cancer cells. In your book you list four different ways that proliferation can be affected. These are: 1) preventing cells from entering the cell cycle, 2) inducing necrosis, (drastic cell death), 3) inducing apoptosis, (natural cell death), and 4) inducing differentiation. Maybe you can say a bit about each of these?

JB: Sure. These are the end effects of what happens on a cellular level after treatment—there are not many things that can happen. In the first, a cell survives but doesn't proliferate—that would be keeping the cell out of the cell cycle. The 'cell cycle' is a term that refers to the machinery set into place when a cell divides. For example, one part of the cell cycle is the process of duplicating its DNA to pass on to the daughter cells. If a cancer cell does not enter the cell cycle, it will not proliferate and will not present much of a problem.

Another end option is that the cell dies of necrosis. You can think of this as an untidy, violent death, perhaps caused by a strong poison, where the outer membrane ruptures before immune cells can ingest the dying cell and the cell's contents spill into the surrounding area. This is not the desired outcome therapeutically, as it has unwanted consequences. One of these is inflammation of the local tissue, which itself can assist in the progression of remaining cancer cells.

A more desirable therapeutic outcome is apoptosis, or programmed cell death. It is a more gentle form of death that is programmed into the cell to occur when conditions are ripe. Like leaves falling from trees in the autumn, it is quite natural. Cells are programmed to undergo apoptosis when it would favour the body as a whole. For example, aged cells should die a peaceful death. In contrast to necrosis, immune cells ingest the apoptotic cell before it has a chance to spill its contents, so no inflammation is produced. Many natural compounds, and some chemotherapy drugs for that matter, can induce apoptosis.

SK: The last end point for a cell is differentiation—can you explain to us about this?

JB: Differentiation is a measure of the degree of maturity of a cell. If a cell is very immature, then it has a strong ability to proliferate. For example, think of the cells that exist in a growing foetus soon after conception. They are very immature—they barely resemble the mature skin, or the bone, or the heart cells later seen in the child. They are still very pliable, able to proliferate quickly and mature into a variety of different tissues. At the other extreme are fully differentiated cells. A brain cell is a good example. It has completely lost its ability to proliferate—it just lives out its life and then dies.

Some cancer cells are poorly differentiated. For example, some cells from a breast cancer may barely resemble the cells from normal breast tissue. But some natural compounds can induce such cells to mature—turning them into cells that more closely resemble the tissue from which they came. In the process, proliferation is reduced.

SK: Before we end I would like to talk about the dosage estimates you have calculated. Personally, I consider they are extraordinarily significant. For instance—taking quercetin as an example—you have calculated that a required dose might be between 0.25 and 1.8 grams per day, if synergism is present. This is a major step forward toward logical use of these compounds therapeutically.

JB: I believe my book is the first attempt to systematically estimate the doses that might be required for clinical effect. However, it is just a first attempt, and the estimates are only ballpark figures designed to guide further research—crude approximations from models I was able to design. But nonetheless, they are probably the best estimates that are available because before this the issue has hardly been addressed at all.

And while we're on this clinical topic—I would like to emphasize that my book is not intended as a self-treatment guide. But I do hope it will provide useful and enlightening material for conversations between patients and healthcare providers. Cancer is a very complex disease and I believe patients are best served by working with a multi-talented team of professionals. I have very little clinical experience myself; primarily I'm a researcher. So whatever I have to say has to be blended with opinions from those who have clinical experience, as well as opinions from other researchers.

SK: In this book, we have tried to emphasize to the reader that they would do best if they locate an appropriate professional to work with. I should add that your web site (www.ompress.com) has some resources that might help them locate one.

John, we have covered all I had planned—so I would like to thank you for everything you have so clearly explained.

JB: Thank you as well.

Diet / Food Choice – Metabolic Typing

Metabolic Typing is about making the food you eat work in same way as beneficial medicine. In fact, the right food for your metabolic type is probably just as powerful as any medication you can take.

The reason we are presenting Metabolic Typing rather than one of the many other 'cancer diets', is because it identifies foods that act as beneficial medicine for *each individual's* metabolic type—rather than proscribing 'blanket recommendations' regardless of individual metabolic functioning.

Moreover, it is an easy diet to fit into everyday life. Whichever type you are, it will be possible for you to eat conventional foods, even when going out for a meal.

———————

In comparison with today's usual dietary recommendations, Metabolic Typing seems almost blasphemous. It is quite possible, (after testing), you could come out as a Metabolic Type recommended to eat plenty of rich meat proteins and high quality fats and oils. However, you might come out a different Metabolic Type—for example, one recommended to eat less protein and a higher proportion of carbohydrates in your diet.

Dietary principles such as these startle many doctors and nutritionists. In conventional terms, it is not recommended anybody eat plenty of rich meat protein, fats and oils. But Dr Kelley, and more recently Bill Wolcott, have used Metabolic Typing principles to treat tens of thousands of individuals working to heal themselves of cancer—and much success has been reported.

Metabolic Typing first came to prominence when Dr Gonzalez, of New York, studied and verified many of Kelley's original Metabolic Typing case histories. After looking through Kelley's case records, Dr Gonzalez was amazed to find documentation of many successful treatments. This inspired him to produce a five hundred-page report following up and analysing many of the cases. Dr Gonzalez's report is important because it indicates that following a Metabolic Typing program can be an effective treatment for cancer.

What is Metabolic Typing and where did it originate?

The Metabolic Typing theory of cancer was devised by Dr Kelley. Two life experiences of Dr Kelley's are often cited as the inspiration for the theory. The first experience took place when Dr Kelley himself contracted pancreatic cancer. Pancreatic cancer is one of the severest cancers and has a very low survival rate. However, Dr Kelley treated himself as a vegetarian and recovered.

The second experience involves an illness suffered by Dr Kelley's wife. She became seriously ill after inhaling toxic paint fumes, and as Dr Kelley nursed her, he found there was nothing he could do to improve her condition. Though he treated her as a vegetarian, she became more ill. Eventually it occurred to Dr Kelley that he had not tried giving his wife high levels of meat protein to eat. Kelley therefore began feeding his wife plenty of protein, and it is reported she started to respond and was soon fully recovered. This experience provided Dr Kelley with the spark of insight needed to create the theory of Metabolic Typing.

Dr Kelley initially based Metabolic Typing analysis upon the analysis of a person's ANS (Autonomic Nervous System). However we should note that over recent decades, Metabolic Typing analysis has been improved and enhanced by Bill Wolcott (Kelley's assistant for eight years). Since 1986, Wolcott's Metabolic Typing has been based on the analysis of nine fundamental elements of the body's functioning, rather than on the single element of the ANS. For instance, one of the other nine fundamental elements included in Wolcott's Metabolic Type analysis is 'Blood Type' (present day exponent, Peter D'Adamo – www.dadamo.com)—and it is recommended therefore that a person avoid foods that do not agree with their 'Blood Type' as *part* of their Metabolic Typing program.

As part of his explanation of cancer, Kelley drew on John Beard's theory of cancer (see p.238). Beard's theory states that the pancreas secretes enzymes directly into the blood stream, which in turn protects against cancer by 'dissolving' the outer layer of 'invisible' trophoblast cancer cells. Once the outside layer of trophoblast cancer cells is dissolved, they become visible (and open to attack and destruction) by the immune system. This is at odds with traditional immune system thinking, as it is considered that immune system white blood cells are responsible for dealing with cancer calls—not enzymes.

In terms of a link between the pancreas, enzymes and 'metabolism', Kelley explained that one of the fundamental balances that must exist for full health to be maintained, is protein metabolism. In fact, for perfect health, not only protein metabolism but also all the different metabolisms of the body need to be in perfect balance and harmony.

Fundamentally, from a Metabolic Typing point of view, to be in balance, all the various metabolisms of the body depend on a correct biochemical balance being present. The question becomes—how can we achieve biochemical balance in the body? The answer Metabolic Typing provides is that to achieve biochemical balance, each person needs to eat foods that are '*chemically*' right for their metabolic type, and consume proteins and carbohydrates in the correct proportions.

Metabolic theory explains that no two humans are exactly the same in constitution and dietary requirements, i.e. no two metabolisms can be balanced in the same way. As it turns out, the old adage that 'one man's food is another's poison' is correct. A diet or nutritional protocol that can heal one person with a particular condition can actually worsen the same condition in another person of a different metabolic type.

For optimal biological and mental functioning every human being needs to discover his or her own unique fuel mixture. This means finding out what their own unique diet should consist of in terms of foods, and also the balance of protein to carbohydrate levels that provide the right 'fuel mixture' for their 'system'.

A common analogy used to describing what 'the right fuel mixture' means— is that of a motor vehicle. As you know, at the garage, you commonly have a choice of several different grades of petrol. Obviously for your car engine to run efficiently, you need to fill up with the right kind of fuel—the one your car was designed to run on. With a car, it's easy to find out the correct fuel mixture— you just look it up in the manufacturer's handbook. For us as human beings the method is slightly different, and there are two main determinants that need to be taken into account.

First is to find out which side of your autonomic nervous system is predominant (Autonomic Type). Second is to find out how quickly your cells burn up nutrients (Oxidative Type). Third is to find out which of these is dominant in terms of influence in the body (Dominant Type).

With regard to which side of your nervous system is predominant, the theory explains that we have two branches coming off our autonomic nervous system (the ANS being the part of our system that is not under our conscious control, and which is responsible for regulating processes like digestion, functioning of the pancreas and other organs, secretion of enzymes and hormones, breathing and heart rate, etc). The two branches of the ANS are known as the sympathetic and the parasympathetic. The reason these two branches are important is that they have nerve fibres reaching into all of our organs, and hence directly affect their functioning.

The two branches of the ANS affect organ functioning because one side of the ANS turns organs on and the other side turn organs off. Organs turned on by the sympathetic side are referred to as sympathetic organs and those turned on by the parasympathetic side are referred to as parasympathetic organs. For example, the stomach's secretion of hydrochloric acid is switched on by parasympathetic nerve fibres and turned off by sympathetic nerve fibres. Heartbeat, on the other hand, is increased by sympathetic nerve fibres and slowed by parasympathetic nerve fibres.

Certain foods and nutrients have been found to stimulate the sympathetic side while others stimulate the parasympathetic side. Thus it is important to find out exactly which system is dominant in a person or whether a person is what is known as a balanced type, where both branches are equally developed in terms of their influence.

Therefore the three main categories individuals divide into are:

1   Sympathetic dominant

2   Balanced type

3   Parasympathetic dominants

It is worth noting there is no best type—one is not better than another. Rather, each type has different dietary requirements and consuming the right foods (and dietary mix) will cause each 'types' metabolism to function efficiently—and so promote health. In contrast, providing the wrong mix will cause metabolism to go out of balance and therefore leave an individual at greater risk of illness.

The thrust of MT is to balance body chemistry and maximize metabolic efficiency *within one's genetic metabolic design limit.* Specifically, as mentioned, in terms of cancer the resulting imbalance affects pancreatic functioning, and the optimal secretion of pancreatic enzymes.

The second major category of metabolic functioning is known as 'Oxidative Type' and individuals fall into the following categories:

1   Slow oxidisers

2   Mixed oxidisers

3   Fast oxidisers

A slow oxidiser refers to an individual whose cells burn nutrients and glucose slowly, whereas a fast oxidiser means that body cells utilise nutrients and glucose much more quickly. The mixed type lies somewhere in the middle.

The two main categories (autonomic and oxidative) tend to work in harmony with each other, so that a sympathetic type will tend to be a slow oxidiser and a parasympathetic type will tend to be a fast oxidiser.

However, there is also another variable that needs to be defined by Metabolic Type testing—and is known as 'Dominant Type'. Dominant Type refers to which of the two main categories (autonomic or oxidative) is dominant in its effect upon organ functioning.

Specifically, is it the sympathetic/parasympathetic component, or the fast/slow oxidiser component which is dominant upon an individuals metabolism? This more subtle understanding of metabolism will further influence the diet and therapeutic program followed. The general implications for diet are as follows:

- Sympathetic/slow oxidiser types fare much better on carbohydrates and a lower intake of oils and proteins.

- Parasympathetic/fast oxidisers do better on a high protein, fat and oil intake, with a lower carbohydrate content to their diet.

- Balanced types fall somewhere in the middle.

Based on initial testing, suitable ratios of proteins, fats and carbohydrates are worked out for each individual. This is further refined as the program continues, until the correct 'fuel mix' is established. Also, the fuel mixture required by the body can change throughout the day. Even within the same metabolic type category, there can be significant differences in the macro nutrient ratio required between breakfast, lunch, and dinner. These fluctuations need to be identified for optimum healing and health.

Following the Metabolic Typing program can also involve a program of cleansing and detoxification and individuals are recommended supplements appropriate for their type.

In conclusion, if we compare the approach of Metabolic Typing with that of chemotherapy or radiation, we can note that healing is carried out with food alone, and not with any toxic medications. Even so, as mentioned above, Dr Gonzalez case study report showed exceptional results for difficult-to-cure cancers such as pancreatic cancer.[27]

How to Use Metabolic Typing

The easiest service to use is run by the company Healthexcel (an internet search will bring up Healthexcel approved practitioners). Healthexcel offer several levels of testing, some for individuals already experiencing good health who want to identify their metabolic type, and other programs more suitable for individuals with a serious health condition.

The level specifically recommended for individuals with a serious health condition is the Advanced Program (though it is possible to start with the simpler Intermediate Program (which is questionnaire based only) if you wish. The Advanced Program has a first phase spaced over month and begins with a series of home tests carried out over the first four days.

The tests are straightforward and can be carried out easily by most people, though a bit of help from a friend or relative is useful. The tests consist of glucose and potassium challenge tests (i.e. your body's response to a specified amount of glucose and potassium) along with timed measurements of saliva pH, urine pH, blood pressure, temperature and heart rate. A comprehensive questionnaire covers all aspects of your physiology and general responses to food and other important factors. Experience has shown it is possible to predict individuals' metabolic types from questionnaires almost as accurately as from physiological tests. However for the advanced test as much individual data as possible is gathered using both a questionnaire and practical tests.

After you have completed the home tests and questionnaire, the data is submitted via the internet and analysed by a computer program. The results of the analysis will include details of your individual metabolic type, details of a suitable starting diet and a list of suitable supplements. Your MT advisor will be on hand to help you understand exactly what your results mean, and how they should be translated into meals that are right for your metabolism.

Approximately two weeks after starting the diet, you will carry out a brief mid-way test to check your metabolism is responding. Later, at the month point, you will carry out a complete retest (i.e. the same tests carried out at the beginning of the month). This will provide an indication of how you are responding, and whether any corrections to your diet need to be made. As you continue longer term, diet sheets will monitor how you are feeling after meals and again analysis of these will allow small but important adjustments to be made to your diet until, eventually, you arrive at a detailed and practical understanding of your metabolic requirements.

Where to go for more information: http://www.healthexcel.com or do an internet search for 'Metabolic Typing' or 'Metabolic Type Diet'.

Cost: In terms of cost, presuming you need to purchase testing equipment such as a blood pressure gauge, glucose meter or thermometer—the following figures are a rough guide.

Item	Approx cost
Cost of testing items	£90 ($144)
Cost of advanced program*	£240 ($384)
Approx cost of suggested supplements	£150 ($240) /month

* This cost includes the two full tests, a midway test and one hair analysis. Further tests will be subject to additional fees

Table 7: Approximate 1st Month Metabolic Typing Costs

Interview With Bill Wolcott (Metabolic Typing)

Bill Wolcott is Kelley's former assistant and founder of Healthexcel, an organisation offering Metabolic Typing assessments to the general public.

Simon Kelly: Bill, thank you for your time today. To start with, with reference to Metabolic Typing, I am wondering if you can give us an indication of the number of people you have advised over the years?

Bill Wolcott: Thank you, it is a pleasure. I would say, between Dr Kelley and myself, it has to be well over sixty thousand people.

SK: And of those sixty thousand individuals, how many were working to heal themselves of cancer?

BW: I would estimate that between a third to a half of them were suffering from cancer. However in the Metabolic Typing approach we don't really differentiate whether a person has cancer or diabetes, arthritis, chronic fatigue or any other health problem.

It makes no difference to us what illness a person is suffering from because we have learned that diseases are in fact, the symptoms. That is, diseases are not the real problem, rather they're the expression of underlying imbalances—the same way that waves on the ocean are visible on the surface, yet their cause is down deep within the ocean itself. The same is true with diseases of the body—diseases are the symptoms, the outer expressions of imbalances and inefficiencies in the body's fundamental control systems.

Therefore we don't treat the disease directly. In fact, two individuals with the *same* disease may be put on totally different, totally opposite biochemical protocols—each of which is correct for *their* particular Metabolic Type. To get people well—all we focus on is their individual Metabolic Type. That is, what balances *their* body chemistry… what detoxifies *their* body…

In a very real sense, we do not treat cancer… we treat *the person* who has cancer. In Metabolic Typing, we always treat the person who has the disease rather than the disease that has the person.

Through Metabolic Tying we are able to balance body chemistry, maximize metabolic efficiency and restore factors that were previously missing—factors such as optimal energy production in the cell. Restoring these missing biochemical factors allows cells to properly fulfil their activities—whatever they may be. All cells (brain cells, liver cells, kidney cells, immune cells, etc) are dependent on the proper biochemical balance being present for optimal function—and through Metabolic Typing, we have discovered that different individuals have different genetically-based food and nutrient requirements.

SK: In terms of providing cells with the nutrients they need, I have always imagined that cells float around in a kind of a soup—and that the soup contains various nutrients that cells can take up and absorb. Also, I always thought the main fuel for the cell is just simple glucose?

BW: Well, this is a great point because I think many people also share this perception of cells just being this big conglomeration in the body soup. But that is very, very far from the reality.

The body is structured in a very hierarchical and organized manner. At the top level, (the most complex level), is the organism as a whole. But that organism is comprised of various systems: the digestive system, the cardio-vascular system, the immune system and so forth. In turn, these systems are comprised of various organs and glands—and the organs and glands are comprised of various tissues. The tissues are comprised of cells. And the cells are built upon the nucleus—and then there are the sub-nucleus levels.

These different levels are separated through membranes into different compartments—and at each level there needs to be very specific balances of certain nutrients present. If the necessary nutrients are absent, then there will be a problem at that particular level in the body.

In terms of the cell itself and its utilisation of fuel, yes glucose is taken into the cell, but the functioning and the utilisation of that is dependent upon cellular processes called glycolysis, the citric acid cycle (or Krebs cycle) and beta oxidation.

These are the processes that run the energy production in cells. Of great importance is the fact that each of these processes has a number of steps within them, and in turn, *each of the steps requires very specific nutrients*. If these nutrients are lacking, then it uncouples or it disrupts that particular aspect of the energy production and the cell will be incapable of producing the energy needed for its proper functioning.

This is where we get into metabolic individuality. For example, one Metabolic Type category that we recognise is known as Oxidative Type. What we call a 'Fast Oxidiser' is an individual that has a metabolism with stronger glycolysis activity and weaker beta oxidation. In contrast, the 'Slow Oxidiser' Metabolic Type has weaker glycolysis and stronger beta oxidation. As a result, Fast Oxidizers burn carbohydrates too quickly and therefore need a diet high in protein and fat to bring the energy-producing systems into balance. Conversely, Slow Oxidizers do poorly on a diet high in fat and protein, and need to eat a much higher percentage of carbohydrates (e.g. fruits, vegetables, grains) in order to maximize their energy production.

This is why diet is so important—because the foods and nutrients we consume fuel the processes of energy production within the cell—glycolysis, the citric acid cycle and beta-oxidation. The important point to note is that if we cannot get the right balance of nutrients for our particular genetic makeup, then the whole machinery of energy production is uncoupled and becomes dysfunctional.

When this happens, the cell is not able to produce the energy it needs to fulfil its activity. And of course, when you have cellular dysfunction then you have organ or gland dysfunction, because the cells comprise the organs and the glands.

For instance, if you have a group of liver cells that are dysfunctional, maybe you then have a dysfunctional liver. And in turn, if you have a dysfunctional liver, then you have a dysfunctional system—a dysfunctional system of elimination and detoxification.

SK: It sounds like you're saying, 'focus first on the functioning of one single body cell'. A cell sounds a very simple thing but actually it's an incredibly complex phenomenon.

BW: Yes. Let's consider the question—'Where does our energy come from?' Our energy has to come from somewhere. How does the body live from day to day? How do we have the energy to get up off of our chair, eat breakfast, go to work, and carry out all of the other things we do?

That energy is being generated within the body. But where in the body? Of course it is within the cells. Each of those hundred trillion cells that form the body is producing energy, and that energy is being used to run the body.

As the machinery of the body, if your heart needs to pump faster, then heart cells have to work harder at what they do. In order to do that they need to be able to produce more energy. If they can't produce the energy they need, then the efficiency of the heart cells is deficient—and that makes the heart activity itself deficient.

So there's always this hierarchy based upon the foundation of energy production that takes place in all cells of the body. That's why nutrition is so important and why metabolic individuality is so important—because different people need different kinds of fuel to run the engines of metabolism that we call the cells. Thus not only is there no one diet that is right for everyone, there is no one treatment for *any* given disease that is effective for all people with that disease. That is what metabolic individuality is all about and why Metabolic Typing—matching foods and nutrients to an individual's metabolism—is so important.

Remember what I described earlier about the two Oxidative Types—the Fast and Slow Oxidisers. In order to be healthy, each individual type *must* eat according to the requirements of their particular kind of metabolism. Lets consider an example. Imagine two people, one a Slow Oxidizer and the other a Fast Oxidizer, are both suffering with heart disease. In our system, the Slow Oxidiser would be placed on a high carb, low fat, low protein protocol and the Fast Oxidiser on the biochemical opposite—a high protein, high fat, low carb protocol. *Yet both would get well.*

We have seen this thousands of times with all manner of degenerative conditions. This is what I meant when I said that you can't treat the disease; rather you must treat the individual, the Metabolic Type, the person who has the disease. Amazingly, this is true for any condition, whether it be heart disease, cancer, arthritis or any other degenerative condition you can think of.

SK: That makes me think of the notion of the average balanced diet. In our society, the recommended balanced diet contains a certain fixed percentage of proteins, carbohydrates, fats and oils. Doesn't this kind of balanced diet cover all the cell's requirements—isn't there enough leeway in every organism so that an average 'balanced diet' is sufficient in terms of nutrients for everyone?

BW: Well in a sense, yes. People can live, they can survive, but that doesn't mean that they will be healthy and living in 'optimal health'. Look at the United Sates and Europe. A lot of people are suffering from degenerative diseases, and with each subsequent generation, we are seeing these 'diseases of the aged', in younger and younger people. I mean, children never used to have heart disease, high cholesterol, arterial sclerosis and diabetes, but now they are becoming commonplace in young people.

So yes, people can survive on any type or ratios of protein, carbohydrate and fat, but not in an optimal way. The body cannot maintain itself at an 'optimal' level because it may be getting the wrong kind of fuel for its 'engines of metabolism'. The eventual result of this situation will be a degenerative process that if left unchecked will become a full blown, diagnosable degenerative disease.

This goes back to ancient history. It goes back to thinking about how peoples throughout the world populated the globe. People settled in the Arctic, people settled in the tropical climates… People settled in every nook and cranny on the planet.

Up until a couple of hundred years ago, people didn't have jet travel and cars to zoom around the globe. Wherever you were born, you pretty much stayed until your death. So generation after generation lived in the circle of local environments where only certain kinds of foods were available. Through the processes of natural selection, genetic mutation and survival of the fittest, only those individuals who could thrive on the kind of food available locally lasted through the generations.

Those who were born unsuited for the particular type of food available in their local environment—those were the 'weak' ones. Those were the ones who couldn't run fast enough to get away from the wolf or the tiger. Those were the ones who couldn't win the knife fight. We know that for the most part, survival of the fittest weeds the 'weak' out of the genetic pool. These are the reasons that Eskimos can live on ten pounds of meat a day, handfuls of fat and no carbohydrate. But if you or I were to eat such a diet, chances are we'd develop cancer, diabetes and heart disease. Yet, until recently, the Eskimos didn't even have a word for cancer in their language.

SK: Just pondering the change, from the beginning of the century, when cancer statistics were approximately one in thirty to the present time, where it's around one in three—it seems confusing because most of us consider our diet is actually much better than it used to be. For the vast majority of people, there is more food available and more variety…

BW: I do not think diet is better now, except calorie-wise. Calories are available to us everyday, whereas in the past this wasn't necessarily the case. However, of most significance is that the *quality* of food today is drastically *worse* than it used to be…

SK: So going back to your previous point, you're saying that we've moved away from consistency. Consistency, in that past generations ate a fairly consistent diet and so over time people's genetic structure became adapted for each regions food. However, now people move around and they travel… there's no consistency anymore.

BW: And the fact that foods from all over the world are available to most people in modern societies.

SK: Like pineapples in the winter over here in the UK.

BW: That's exactly right. Here, in the foothills of the Cascade Mountains our winters are very cold and we have a lot of snow. But in the grocery store—though it's twenty degrees Fahrenheit below zero outside, there are pineapples, strawberries, apples and grapes, shipped in from all over world.

SK: You think we need to pass those by?

BW: Well, I would. What I'm saying is that not only do people have all that, but also all of the junk food, all of the processed food and all of the poor quality food containing large amounts of sugar and fat—fat that has been transformed from its natural state.

It's a two-headed monster. On the one hand we are not eating the foods we are genetically designed to eat and that are right for our Metabolic Type, and on the other hand, we're dealing with the very abhorrent quality of today's food with all its herbicides, pesticides, chemical preservatives and other contaminants. It's reckoned that ten thousand different chemicals have been added to our food supply over the last hundred years. It's an extraordinary thing that has occurred and we are seeing extraordinary adverse effects as a result.

SK: I understand—as you say it is most definitely a double headed monster.

Going back then—linking this with cancer… In terms of metabolic dysfunction, what is it that causes cancer? Metabolic Typing theory specifically mentions dysfunction of the pancreas (and its release of digestive enzymes that dissolve the outer protein layer of trophoblasts—see p.238). Is that view still held or is cancer considered more of a general dysfunction of the immune system?

BW: Well, for us, cancer has always been evidence of extreme degeneration and loss of metabolic efficiency. And yes, in many cases it involves enzyme depletion, because the production of pancreatic enzymes is one of the body's first lines of defence. There's a famous physician by the name of Emanuel Revici…

Revici also saw pancreatic enzyme production as one of the body's early defences. So it's part of the picture, but it isn't the whole picture. The whole picture has to do once again with this domino effect. On the one hand the person who is in good health will, one hundred per cent of the time, resist cancer. Cancer cells may be produced in the body, but they will also immediately be destroyed by the body. The immune system will handle any cellular aberrations that occur. What happens in the diagnosis of cancer is that all the body's defences and metabolic efficiencies which would normally arrest that process are failing. They've degenerated to the point where they are incapable of handling the threat. That allows cancer to grow pretty much at its own will.

But when you balance body chemistry, when you detoxify the body, when you stop doing the wrong things for your Metabolic Type and start doing the right things for your Metabolic Type, then that whole process gets reversed. You start to restore the body's innate capacity to handle any challenge that faces it.

SK: I'm getting an image of health as a sine wave on an oscilloscope—a nice smooth regular up and down sine wave. But illness and disease are more like when the oscilloscope screen is filled with 'noise'—covered in unrelated, inconsistent waveforms.

BW: You know, there's even more to that concept, but that's a very good concept, and an accurate one. If you first picture a sine wave drawn on a piece of paper, where the sign wave is going above and below the central horizontal line in equal portion. What happens in any degenerative disease, including cancer, is that the sign wave is no longer able to go on both sides of the line. It remains stuck on one side, the body's defence is no longer capable of dealing with the other side. The adaptation response to stress fails to resolve the stress.

This can happen in numerous instances. It could be within the autonomic nervous system where you have an excessive sympathetic imbalance and no parasympathetic response, or the reverse. Or you could have this in Revici's approach where you have a catabolic imbalance or an anabolic imbalance.

SK: Anabolic and catabolic—could you explain those terms a little bit more? I'm not really clear what they mean.

BW: Well, the way they are commonly used, catabolic refers to a breaking down process, whereas, anabolic is a building up process. In Revici's system, he found that those activities were also related to very specific biochemistry at the tissue level. He found that the catabolic processes produced aerobic metabolism, and, in terms of the membrane permeability of tissues themselves, it increased the porosity of the membranes. It opened up the membrane.

Anabolic is just the opposite. Anabolic processes produce the anaerobic type of metabolism, the 'without oxygen' type of metabolism. And it also involves a closing down of the cell membranes.

In a healthy individual, the body is able to spontaneously move from aerobic to anaerobic as the situation demands. But when cancer is present, the body becomes stuck in either a catabolic or anabolic mode—it gets stuck in either an aerobic or anaerobic imbalance. Homeostatic activity is lost at the tissue level in terms of the catabolic and anabolic processes, in terms of aerobic and anaerobic activity, in terms of selective membrane permeability, and in terms of pH.

The catabolic imbalances result in alkaline tissue imbalance, and the anabolic imbalances result in acid tissue imbalance. It's always about balance and homeostasis. It is a state of balance where the body can always adapt to a challenge, it can always return to a homeostatic balance in response to a challenge.

Degenerative disease occurs when that sign wave is stuck on one side or the other. It can't respond, it can't adapt to the challenge that is being thrown at it. It doesn't matter what disease we are talking about—it will be true in any degenerative process. There will be imbalances where the body is stuck on one side or other of these fundamental homeostatic controls.

SK: There's a kind of a rigidity to it, isn't there? You've described that the body should have an ability to be responsive, but instead, during times of illness there is rigidity. The body becomes fixed and not able to move or respond.

BW: Correct. Here's a simple analogy or example—temperature. Normally, if temperature rises then the body's adaptation mechanisms spring into play to cool the body down. If the body is too cold, then the opposite process comes into play—to warm the body up. During disease, whether we're talking about autonomic, oxidative, catabolic, anabolic, or any of the fundamental control systems, it is as if the body is stuck on hot regardless of what is happening with the temperature outside—or the body is stuck on cold. It can't change, it can't respond to the challenge that is coming from the environment—in this case, the internal environment.

SK: How do you measure the anabolic and the catabolic flexibility of the body during the Metabolic Typing tests?

BW: Through what we call our circadian test where you check your pH's and specific gravity four times a day. You should cycle above and below the median points. If you don't, then there's a possibility that you're dealing with a catabolic or anabolic imbalance.

But it gets tricky and it's not something you just go off and do on your own because sometimes the imbalance is actually the body's defence. And this opens a whole new can of worms, if you will, a new Pandora's box.

So often, practitioners take lab tests, look at something, let us say the pH, see that it's out of balance, and then begin to treat it. But how do they know what they're looking at? Are they looking at an example of the problem itself? Is the body too acid—or are they looking at the body's defence against the alkalinity? Sometimes you can totally undermine the body's defence against the problem and end up worsening the problem that was there in the first place.

SK: So part of what you are doing in terms of the Metabolic Typing analysis is working out whether any specific measurement is part of the problem or whether it's the body's defence?

BW: That's right.

SK: OK… I want to go back to this idea that Metabolic Typing works at the cellular level…

BW: Metabolic typing works on all levels. It's not restricted to a given level…

SK: OK. But cancer always seems so 'huge'. Somehow it's different from other diseases. Chemotherapy and radiotherapy thrive on this very idea—that to deal with cancer you need something really powerful, and I guess, quite violent.

BW: The approach modern medicine has taken is beyond belief. It defies logic, it defies reason, it defies common sense. Chemotherapy and radiation are always directed toward the tumour, but the tumour is not the cancer—the tumour is the by-product, it's the end product of the disease. Those approaches do nothing to correct the underlying imbalance that allowed cancer to develop in the first place.

It's as if—to take it to its logical absurdity—you look out of your window and notice your apple tree is turning brown. And you think, 'the leaves are brown, well, I better go and paint them green'. So you go out with a can of paint and paint them green. Now you no longer have brown leaves—but what has that done to the cause of the brown leaves? Of course it's done nothing. Or you can think in terms of surgery, you can cut the leaves off— but you still haven't corrected the problem that caused it in the first place—and this is why cancers usually come back.

SK: Bill, I would like to hear about your experience of seeing the body disassemble cancer tumours. As you mentioned you've worked with a lot of people, some twenty to thirty thousand with cancer.

BW: Well, the body, given the opportunity, will destroy the cancer and it will do it in one of two ways. It will either begin to break down and gobble up the tumour, or, it will encapsulate it with a capsule like shell and literally strangle the tumour to death. Once you've corrected the underlying imbalance in the body, the body can handle the condition.

However a mistake many people make (practitioners as well), is that they develop tunnel vision. They decide that cancer is a nutritional problem. So they treat it nutritionally, but then they discover it doesn't seem to help.

That's incredibly short-sighted because there could be multiple factors or multiple causes of the cancer. Remember the various levels I mentioned earlier, organ level, tissue level, cell level, nuclear level and so forth. Diseases will impact or influence one of those levels, but the causal factor can be multiple. It could be nutritional, and if it is nutritional then doing Metabolic Typing will 'miraculously' resolve the condition fairly swiftly.

But there may be other causes. It could be a structural imbalance. It could be an imbalance in the TMJ, (the temporomandibular joint), because the bite impacts the nervous system. It could be a structural imbalance in the cranium, the neck or the spine. It could be heavy metal toxicity. Perhaps a person has accumulated high levels of cadmium, arsenic, lead or mercury. It could be a parasite-based problem. It could be environmental toxins— chemical toxins that have accumulated in the body. It could be electro-magnetic stress. It could even be emotional trauma that has led to the degenerative process.

Nutrition is important and helpful, but you will never resolve or heal the problem with nutrition if the problem itself is caused from a different level other than nutritional. So nutrition is one component and must always be considered, but it is not always the cause.

SK: What you have described there is looking at the problem holistically? Interestingly, working on the emotional level has been shown by certain studies to exert a very beneficial influence over tumour progression (see p.15). It's quite remarkable considering nothing 'physical' is being done.

BW: Many cancers have been cured by working at the emotional level. There have been pioneers in this area and many cancers have been cured by emotional work alone. Of course that's limited as well and failures will occur when the emotional level isn't the causal level. Often when things don't work, it's not that the therapy itself is 'bad'. Certainly there are 'bad' therapies that don't make sense, but in many cases it's not the therapy itself that's bad—it's the fact that the causal factor is different from that being addressed by the therapy being utilised.

SK: You're emphasising the need to look for the causal factor in an individual's illness. In the same vein we could say that you have enlarged Metabolic Typing to include more dimensions—fundamental homeostatic controls as you call them. When I look through the list of fundamental homeostatic controls I get the feeling you've incorporated the best of our understanding of the body—for instance Revici's work mentioned above, as well as others. I'm presuming that Metabolic Typing is not a closed system, and that if more systems of the body are found, and are easily measured, that in the future you will incorporate them.

BW: Very definitely. My feeling is that there will most likely be others.

One of my discoveries has been this idea of causal factors. In my opinion, if you're not searching for the causal factors then you're not asking the right questions. Under the original Kelley program all we looked for was sympathetic or parasympathetic imbalance, and then treated everybody accordingly. A lot of people got well because they happened to have that particular imbalance, but some others didn't get well, and some people got worse than they were before.

It was only by finding other causal factors that happened to be involved in those individuals that we became successful. It has been this search for relevant casual factors that has led to the development and incorporation of the present nine fundamental homeostatic controls into the Healthexcel System of Metabolic Typing.

SK: Your describing that you have researched into making the system work better?

BW: Right, so if it turned out that someone wasn't being helped, then it was time to go back to the drawing board. What am I missing? What is not being addressed by what we are doing? And that's where we uncovered and found out about these other elements. So far we haven't discovered anymore, but I'm just one person and if more people hear about this and get involved, hopefully a lot of great minds will jump into this and carry out more research. Very possibly they will come up with additional elements that are involved. But each one of these levels involves certain nutrients and or certain foods, and they have very precise effects on the particular imbalance of these given levels.

SK: OK. Bill, I want to ask you the following question. If I follow Metabolic Typing, does that stop me from doing other alternative cancer therapies? For instance, you seem to have quite different vitamin C recommendations than Linus Pauling outlines. Sometimes Metabolic Typing seems quite strict.

BW: We have never stated to anyone that you need to do Metabolic Typing and nothing else. I encourage people to bring us ideas or items that they feel would be helpful so we can talk about them and see what impact those particular factors will have on their particular Metabolic Type.

You see for the most part, every nutrient in every food has a pretty specific effect on one or more of these imbalances. So I'm not closed minded, rather I'm saying, 'look, if you want to use vitamin C let's look at your particular metabolism and see what the impact will be for you'. For one person it will have one effect but for another individual it will have a different effect and there are also different forms of vitamin C. One individual can do very well with ascorbic acid but a different individual, because of their acid alkaline imbalance and the fundamental control imbalances that they have, would do much better using something like calcium ascorbate, (a different form of vitamin C) as it has a very different effect of the body. I do not see Metabolic Typing as restrictive, rather I see it as a foundational protocol on which other choices can be made in an intelligent manner.

SK: That sounds more broad and open that I have previously been led to believe. You are saying, 'Let's take a look at how these other therapies impact your biochemistry'.

BW: Well yes, but I think that it's also fair to say that Metabolic Typing is strict in one sense. If you're going to do Metabolic Typing, the primary reason to do it is to find out what is right for you and what is wrong for you. If after this process you turn around and say, 'well I want to do these other things that are wrong for me because I happen to like them'—then don't waste your time with Metabolic Typing. Why even come to us in the first place?

SK: When people have cancer they only have a limited number of hands they can play. They say, 'why not incorporate as many different anticancer therapies as possible'.

BW: Well again, the reason is that some of them may adversely impact body chemistry. Here's a really simple example; there are a number of herbs that are specific for insomnia, but if you take each of those herbs and apply them to an individual who has insomnia, some of those herbs will actually stimulate or create insomnia—i.e. even though they are anti-insomnia herbs, they will have the opposite effect. This is true for any type of therapy. If it's not right for the constitution of the individual, it won't have the desired effect. Instead, it will affect the body on a different level than the intended level.

SK: In terms of incorporating conventional therapies, what is your view about surgery? Quite a few alternative approaches recommend surgery, if only to lower the burden on the body by the removal of cancerous tissue.

BW: We agree with that in general. I ask, is this person strong enough for the surgery? If it's operable, then sure it's a fine thing to do. There's always a risk in surgery. If a person's aware of that and they're willing to do it, then OK, because you are saving the body all the effort, all of the work and all of the time to bring the tumour down cell by cell. Of course surgery does nothing to remove the cause of the cancer.

SK: Removing the tumour can ease the burden on the body and help make space for healing…

BW: I believe that the body is programmed to be healthy, programmed to be perfect and it's constantly trying to do that. It is constantly trying to restore balance within every level. It's only its incapacity to do so that leads to break down and to degeneration. I feel this is our greatest gift and our greatest goal, and is something that every person with a serious illness needs to understand and hold on to.

Like a computer program that is constantly running, the body is always attempting to create perfect health. All we are doing with our approach is giving the body that opportunity. How? By stopping the things that are wrong for it and by doing the things that are right—and by helping the body detoxify whatever toxins are accumulating. If you can do that, you begin to free up the program that has been inhibited in a person's metabolism—the program of health. The body is perfectly capable of restoring health given the opportunity.

SK: Your saying the question is always, 'What's stopping the body healing itself?' I want to ask you now about the detoxification you have mentioned several times. Detoxification is one of the cornerstones of most alternative approaches to health. On a cellular level, how true is the 'process' of detoxification?

BW: Well it's very true. Every cell in the body is programmed and designed to detoxify itself. If it weren't able to detoxify, every cell would die of its own autointoxication—it would literally asphyxiate on its own metabolic waste. All of those cellular metabolic chemical processes we discussed earlier produce metabolic waste. If a cell didn't have a way to move those substances out, waste would over accumulate and poison it.

Remember what we were saying earlier about energy production? If the energy production in a cell is deficient, then it inhibits every activity of the cell—including its ability to detoxify itself. What happens when you reverse that situation—when you restore the energy production to the cell? What happens when you provide the chelating factors necessary to pick up heavy metals and other toxic substances and when you restore selective membrane permeability, so that membranes open to release toxins and close to keep toxins out?

The answer is that when you restore those three things, suddenly the innate capacity of that cell to detoxify kicks into gear. Now there are a hundred trillion little garbage cans starting to mobilise toxins out of the intracellular environment, into the extra-cellular environment. The toxins being dumped by the cells now flood the blood stream. Those toxins are taken to the organs of detoxification to be processed out of the body; the liver, colon, lungs, kidneys and skin. But if these organs are not functioning efficiently, then they act as a bottleneck to the elimination of those toxins from the body.

As a result the toxins back up in the bloodstream just like a sewer when it gets clogged. This is what produces the healing crisis with its sick feeling, aches, pains, fevers, etc. The healing crisis happens because of the restoration of the cellular mobilisation of toxins. This is why we need to regulate the rate of change that takes place—otherwise a person can become very sick from this toxic mobilisation. This is why I refer to balancing body chemistry through Metabolic Typing as the greatest detoxifier.

SK: Bill—thank you for your time and explanations. We explain how readers can contact Healthexcel and organise to have a Metabolic Typing assessment carried out. Thank you very much.

BW: Thank you too. I sincerely appreciate the opportunity to talk about Metabolic Typing.

Photodynamic Therapy (PDT) with Spirulina Based Agent

Photodynamic Therapy (PDT) consists of two components: the first is a special agent that when taken orally, is more attracted to cancer cells than to normal healthy cells. That is, the agent accumulates more in cancer cells than in healthy cells. The second component of PDT is a light source of the correct wavelength. The light source is used to illuminate the areas of the body where cancer is present. As the agent (now present on the inside of cancer cells) is illuminated by the light, it becomes energised—the end result of which, is the formation of singlet oxygen inside cancer cells. Singlet oxygen is a powerful free radical that is able to cause irreversible damage to cells. Ideally the level of damage should be sufficient enough to cause the cells to die, or at least prevent them undergoing any further cell divisions.

You can read more detail about PDT and CLT (Cellular Light Therapy), including information about some clinics that are offering the treatment, in the dedicated section starting p.146. The reason PDT is listed in this section is because over the last year, some much lower cost PDT options have become available—and you may wish to consider incorporating them into your home based program. You will need a light and an appropriate agent. You will find two sources listed below.

One word of caution: so as to proceed as safely as possible you should carry out this treatment under the care of an experienced PDT practitioner. PDT is an emerging and fast changing field, however, the agent manufacturers and suppliers listed below are likely to be able to put you in touch with an appropriate practitioner. Bill Porter of CLT Clinics describes the danger of this therapy, 'because these agents are extremely sensitive to light, it's possible, if treatment isn't done appropriately, that too much agent in combination with too much light could lead to a terrible photochemical burn on the skin'.

Agent & light Suppliers

Operation Hope Clinic (Run by: Professor Noel Campbell) – Offers agent and light for sale to general public.

Clinic: Level 5 167 Collins Street Melbourne Victoria Australia
Correspondence: Post Office Box 137 Parkville VIC 3052 Australia
☎: 03 9639 6090 International 613 9639 6090
🖶: 03 9639 4006 International 613 9639 4006
☎: (Prof. Campbell 0412 994 001 International 61412 994 001)

Email noelc@smile.org.au
Web www.smile.org.au

Cost of agent: £40 ($74) per week.
Light Source: Agent tuned light source is £613 ($1135)

Radapharma public sales:

www.bioresource.biz/
client@bioresource.biz
Elan Group S.A.
Post address: 1108 Budapest, Agyagfejto ut.4, IX/36, Hungary

☎: +36 20 921 9017

Radapharma main site:

http://www.radapharma.ru

Agent name: Photostim

Cost: €250 (£166/$308) for 100ml (lasts between 7–40 days depending on dose taken).

Light source: Best to use the light available from Operation Hope Clinic. Radapharma do sell light sources of their own, but they are rather expensive.

Burzynski's Aminocare A10® Cell Protector

Antineoplastons are compounds that come under the 'chemical' heading of peptides. Originally working to compare substances in the blood and urine of healthy individuals with substances contained in the blood and urine of individuals with cancer, Dr Burzynski noticed an important difference. Specifically he identified that individuals with cancer are low on antineoplastons. Years of research (and therapeutic use of antineoplastons) has identified that antineoplastons form part of the body's communication system—a system it uses to instruct cells to turn *off* any 'cancerous growth'.

You can read about Burzynski's antineoplastons in more detail in the Group 3 Therapies section (including an interview with Dr Burzynski)—see p.119.

Until recently, antineoplastons have only been available at his clinic based in Houston, Texas. However, Dr Burzynski has recently obtained FDA approval to market a lower dose version of his broad spectrum A10 antineoplaston. The supplement contains 49% A10 along with other essential amino acids involved in antineoplaston manufacture within the body.

Though Burzynski makes it clear that this supplement is not a substitute for his intensive antineoplaston cancer therapy treatment, he does suggest it is useful as a complimentary therapy—for instance it has been shown to decrease toxicity associated with chemotherapy.

The supplement contains the following active ingredients:

- A10 (main ingredient making up 49.0% of supplement)

- Additional ingredients: L-Arginine, L-Alanine, Glycine, L-Ornithine, L-Serine, L-Threonine, L-Valine, Ryboflavin

Cost: Aminocare A10 can be ordered directly over the internet and works out at £75 ($120) dollars per month. (Recommended dose: two to four tablets per day).

How to order: You can order Aminocare from: www.volmed.com

Pancreatic Enzyme supplementation

You may remember that enzymes were listed in John Boik's list of recommended compounds. In addition, several other anti-cancer therapies stress the role of pancreatic enzymes, as they purport the protein outer layer of cancer cells is broken down (which in turn renders them visible to the body's immune system), not by immune system killer cells, but by enzymes circulating in the blood stream.

There is some compelling evidence as to the importance of the role enzymes play in the body. In a developing foetus, if its pancreas does not begin excreting pancreatic enzymes exactly on time (the 56th day after conception), then both baby and mother are liable to contract one of the most virulent forms of cancer known—choriocarcinoma. The reason being, enzymes are needed to curtail the action of certain cells (trophoblast cells) which are responsible for carving a niche for the embryo in the wall of the womb in the initial days after conception.

You can read more about the theory behind the use of pancreatic enzymes in the section on John Beard's Trophoblastic Theory of Cancer (p.238).

Cost and how to obtain the therapy:

Enzyme therapy should consist of concentrated pancreatic enzymes as well as proteolytic (protein digesting) enzymes such as papain (from papaya) and bromelain (from pineapple). The main pancreatic enzyme (pancreatin) will automatically include other enzymes such as chymotrypsin, trypsin, lipase, amylase etc, though in some brands these will be added as separate ingredients as well. The enzymes should be taken on an empty stomach—some one to two hours before food.

We recommend enzymes from Life Extension Foundation (see www.lef.org/newshop/items/item00306.html for details) or those produced by Rocky Fork Formulas Inc, specifically their formula marketed under the name of 'Megazyme Forte's. This formula is enteric coated and has 45mg of available chymotrypsin per tablet—as well as all the other necessary enzymes.

Rocky Fork Formulas Inc. can be found at www.rockyfork.net though they do not supply direct. They will help you locate a local supplier—and/or you can do a search on the internet for 'Megazyme Forte'. Here is an example supplier of 'Megazyme Forte'—price is £25.60 ($41) for two hundred tablets (recommended consumption three tablets three times per day):

http://shop.store.yahoo.com/healthgenesis/zyme48.html

Another tried and tested formula is Wobenzym N, though this has considerably less chymotrypsin per tablet (1mg). To find tablets you can carry out an internet search for Wobenzym. Here are some examples of suppliers—price is £18.75 ($30) for two hundred tablets (recommended consumption—three tablets twice daily):

www.buywobenzym.com and www.lef.org

Though many sources claim 'enteric coated' enzymes are important (i.e. a special coating that allows the enzymes to pass through the stomach in an encapsulated form), Dr Gonzalez (a medical doctor presently running a study looking at power of enzymes against cancer) disagrees. He considers 'pork enzymes' such as those sold by the Life Extension Foundation are the best for individuals to take. Read an article about Dr Gonzalez's work with cancer here:

www.lef.org/magazine/mag2003/feb2003_report_acam_01.html

We should note that some cancer practitioners suggest taking between forty to sixty tablets a day—rather than the recommendations listed above. This is because pancreatic enzymes are seen as crucial to the unmasking of cancer cells. It also illustrates that pancreatic enzymes are extremely safe and non-toxic.

Lastly, it is worth noting that Dr Kelly, the originator of Metabolic Typing, recommends that our intake of daily protein be eaten within a period of six hours during the day. This, he contends, frees the enzymes in the body from purely digestive tasks and allows them to work for the other eighteen hours in the day on the outer layer of any potential cancerous trophoblast cells (thus rendering them visible to the immune system).

Gaston Naessens Somatid Therapy and 714-X

Introductory note: The Somatid theory asserts, that for millions of years, human beings have lived in a *symbiotic* relationship with a particular microorganism living in our blood and lymph fluid. In true symbiotic form, this microorganism carry's out useful functions for us (for example, the microorganism appears to be responsible for clotting our blood at the necessary time), and in return we carry out useful functions for it, i.e. provide a host environment. When humans are in good health and the interior environment of the body is as it should be, the symbiotic relation works well for both parties. However, if our internal environment degrades and becomes inhospitable for the microorganism, then the symbiotic relationship breaks down and the microorganism mutates into more advanced forms—which in the end become parasitic to the body and sap our vital ife energy.

Describing the existence of this microorganism is one thing, seeing an actual video of them is another. For this reason we have uploaded a video clearly showing the existence of the somatids existing in live blood to the book linked website.

You can locate the video at: www.healing-cancer.co.uk/resources

The treatment Gaston Naessens has developed (714-X) is particularly worthy of discussion because it is focussed on the lymphatic system. Unhindered functioning of the lymphatic system is as vital for health as the blood circulatory system, however, surprisingly few treatments focus their attention on it. Though for the most part undocumented in their efficacy, other treatment modalities that focus on improving the functioning of the lymphatic system are ozone steam sauna (see p.24) and Light Beam Generator treatments (www.lightbeam-generator.com).

Gaston Naessens' theory is the most recent formulation of a phenomenon that has been observed by various distinguished researchers for over a hundred years (starting with Prof Antoine Beachamp in 1883 and Professor Dr. Gunter Enderlein in 1916). If these men's observations and theories are correct then in time much of our understanding of the life sciences will need reassessing.

Naessens' theory revolves around a new life form he has observed using a special microscope he designed and built himself. Naessens' has named this new life form a 'somatid'. Somatids are extraordinarily small, and there are millions of them in our blood, as well as in the blood of animals and in the sap of plants. Using 'live blood' microscopy techniques, the somatids can be observed and appear like a galaxy of stars glimmering in the night sky.

Naessens considers that the somatids are a crucial element in blood. Experiments have demonstrated that they are somehow related to cellular division and cellular repair, and that they function to sustain life.

How did Naessens discover the somatids?

Naessens discovered the presence of the somatids after he designed his own special microscope which he has called a somatoscope. The observation of somatids is something that was made possible because the somatoscope is superior in terms of its resolving power (i.e. the resolution of the image). With the somatoscope much smaller particles are visible (100 to 150 Angstroms) than with conventional light microscopes. Also the somatoscope permits observation of live material. This is particularly important in terms of somatids, because they need a liquid environment to express themselves. On dry blood smears (dead material) we do not see them—they are invisible.

Even though an electron microscope can magnify in the range of 400,000 to 600,000 times, specimens viewed have to be dehydrated and therefore dead. When it comes to viewing live specimens, at this time nothing can quite match Gaston Naessens' somatoscope. The Somatoscope offers a chance for us to look deeper into the workings of life, just as the Hubble space telescope allows us to look deeper into the depths of space.

(Technical note: For those who are interested in how the somatoscope works, we can explain that the basis of its operation is the combination of two light sources of different wavelengths—processed through a Kerr cell—creating a third light with a shorter wavelength.[28] The shorter wavelength provides more resolving power, which in turn permits better vision of smaller particles. Therefore, by mixing different wavelengths of light and processing them using electromagnets and various filters, an invisible light is created that yields far greater resolution of specimens than is capable with visible spectrum light.)

Over recent years, using the somatoscope, Naessens has studied the somatid life form in detail. He has produced video footage of these life forms, so that other researchers can examine them and also begin to understand their significance.

Further, in recent years Naessens has designed a special diachromic condenser that can be fitted to most contemporary light microscopes. With a microscope fitted with this condenser, any person who wishes to, can clearly see the somatids and the various forms through which they evolve. The condenser is said to have excellent performance, though the design is very different from the somatoscope. (The diachromatic condenser is available from Cerbe Distribution Inc in Canada).

The relationship between somatids & health

It has been observed that when somatids are functioning normally, they go through a three-stage lifecycle. However, before and during times of illness the number of somatid stages changes. Once they have moved from the normal three-stage lifecycle, they can pass through any number—up to a maximum of sixteen different lifecycles.

It should be noted, however, that somatids are 'witnesses' of internal disharmony rather than the actual cause of disharmony. Naessens explains that when the chemistry of the internal body is functioning properly, the somatids are seen in a three-stage life cycle (micro-cycle). But when the immune system starts to be challenged, is weak, or suppressed, then the somatids are seen in their macrocycle—that is, through their sixteen stage life-cycle.

Naessens, with the help of various doctors, has done many years of fieldwork to correlate the somatid stages found in patients' live blood analysis with their actual state of health. From his analysis, Naessens has found that there is a 'gate control' present between stage three and stage four of the somatid lifecycle. In a healthy state the gate is strong, but if a person's immune system begins being deficient, then the gate starts to collapse, until it is fully down. (The purpose of the gate is to restrict somatids to just a three stage life-cycle).

Somatids are described as being pleomorphic (meaning they can change into more and more complex life forms). This clashes with conventional science because the mere existence of pleomorphic life forms has been a particularly contentious point in science for the last hundred years. Science has been supportive of the monomorphic theory for more than a century and most research today is based on the notion that a life form is fixed and constant, and cannot change from one form to another.

The main difference between these two systems is that those individuals, largely influenced by Pasteur, who support monomorphism, insist that a life form is fixed and cannot change form during its life-cycle. For example, a bacteria is a bacteria and it never changes. The other group, pleomorphists, influenced more by Antoine Béchamp, insists on the fact that some life-forms do change form during their life-cycle. For example, a double spore can change into a bacterial-like form. (We ourselves have observed video footage from Naessens showing a somatid changing from one life form to another, and though we cannot claim to be experts in the field, the footage was very clear and convincing—or at least demanded a good answer from supporters of monomorphism).

Over the last century there has been enormous antagonism between the two camps. However, Naessens proposes building a bridge and feels this would lead to us gaining greater insight into diseases such as cancer. His position is that some life structures do behave monomorphically, while others, like the somatids, do without any doubt behave pleomorophically.

The question Naessens has asked himself is how could his discovery of pleomorphic changes of the somatids (as a witness of a suppressed immune system) help individuals overcome cancer? Utilising what he has observed, Naessens has designed a therapy to improve health and, if possible, prevent illness from occurring in the first place.

Naessens has strived to find a non-toxic way to make somatids return to the first three stages of their lifecycle (micro-cycle phase 1-2-3). To this extent he has developed a compound which he has named 714-X. 714-X is injected by individuals themselves, directly into their groin lymph nodes and is thought to work at several levels. First of all, it is often suggested that it liquefies the lymph fluid and helps ease any congestion occurring within the lymph system. (Good flow of lymph fluid is essential for efficient body detoxification).

Secondly, 714-X contains large amounts of nitrogen. This is important because cancer cells are known to be hungry for nitrogen and, in their search for it, send out chemicals that paralyse the host's immune system. The strategy of 714-X is that by satisfying cancer cells' hunger for nitrogen, it will prevent them releasing immune system paralysing compounds—which in turn will free up the immune system to again seek out and destroy cancerous cells.

Thirdly, 714-X supplies a whole range of bio-available trace minerals to the lymphatic system. Naessens' strategy is that by improving the body's overall functioning, particularly that of the lymph system, the 'control gate' will again be put in place by the body—and thus again limit the somatids to just a three stage life-cycle.

In summary, then, let us state the implications of what Naessens is describing to us. The implications are that there is a whole new dimension of 'physical' life operating below the cellular mechanisms of DNA. Naessens is suggesting that if we want to 'cure' disease and illness, then we need to be working at this deeper layer, rather than at the cellular level. Specifically, we need to work to move the somatids back to their normal three-stage cycle. 714-X is the compound that Naessens has developed to help achieve this.

Further we should note Naessens considers the most important implication of his work, is that live blood analysis (specifically the identification of somatid life cycle stages) can act as a unique diagnostic and disease prevention tool. Naessens has observed that somatids start living through a larger number of life cycle stages at least a couple of years before the onset of illness. Thus an alert before disease strikes gives an individual the time and chance to address issues around their health.

714-X is something you can obtain and use at home. It is reasonably low cost, *completely* non-toxic and can be used in conjunction with other health-building therapies (though it is recommended that vitamin B12 and vitamin E are avoided during the actual times you are using 714-X).

Using 714-X as a cancer therapy

As described above, Gaston Naessens produces a substance called 714-X. Naessens has developed 714-X to help the somatids return to a three-stage life cycle.

It is recommended 714-X be taken over a twenty-one-day cycle, with a rest gap between each cycle. 714-X needs to be injected into the groin lymph nodes, and Naessens has produced a video explaining exactly how this should to be done. The aim of the video is to provide enough instruction for you to feel confident enough to self-administer 714-X. However for those who feel they need more intensive face-to-face tuition, short training courses are regularly run in Quebec, Canada.

Injecting the groin lymph nodes sounds frightening, but actually it is very straightforward and virtually pain free. The thought of it is far worse than the reality. In practice the needles are so thin they can hardly be felt—though the camphor (one of the ingredients of 714-X) may sting a little.

Cost: The cost of the therapy is £187.50 ($300) for a twenty-one day supply of the lymphatic system treatment.

How to obtain the therapy: The internet is the best way to make contact with Naessens supply company, Cerbe. The website address is www.cerbe.com

Similar blood normalisation therapies: As mentioned at the beginning of this section the Somatid phenomena has been studied by researchers prior to Naessens. They also developed therapies to address the mutation of somatids into advanced forms. The most noteworthy of these are the Sanum formulations, which are in effect inoculation type formulas. Sanum representatives at www.pleosanum.com will be able to direct you to a practitioner of this therapy in your area.

Obtaining an analysis of your blood: Even without Naessens somatoscope (i.e. his extra powerful microscope), it is possible to view the microorganism that exists in your blood—and any stages it may have mutated to. Start with a search on the internet for a practitioner in your area offering live blood microscopy.

In terms of analysis and interpretation of blood, very few practitioners use the Somatidian framework we have discussed, but quite a few do use Gunter Enderlein's framework of pleomorphism—which is very similar and just as insightful.

Practitioners may also be able to prescribe you the appropriate Sanum formulations (see above for explanation).

Location of Somatid video: www.healing-cancer.co.uk/resources

Q & A With Gaston and Jacinte Naessens (714-X)

Question: How did you come up with the idea of the somatoscope, and the methods used to manipulate the light in this special way?

Answer: Well, there are two ways to improve the resolving power (the quality and resolution of the image), of a light microscope. Both based on the mathematical formula that we use to work out the final resolving power.

One way is to work on the objectives (i.e. the lenses), and improve their numerical aperture for better performance. However, the microscopy industry has brought this to its fullest capacity—and had done so even in the 1950's.

The other way to improve the resolving power of a microscope, is to shorten the wavelength of the visible light source. This is what we have focused on because the microscope industry had not worked on this aspect at all. The reason being that the scientific community contends that it is not possible to go beyond the wavelength of visible light—and they have not been willing to challenge this paradigm [this way of looking at things].

Question: Can the somatoscope's resolving power be further improved and is this something you are working on?

Answer: The somatoscope could always be improved by changing the internal parts for new ones, for instance, more modern lenses. But we have decided to invest our efforts designing new universal condensers that other researchers in the world can fit onto their microscopes. In 2000, we brought out a newly designed diachromic condenser making it easy for others to observe cells and somatid functioning.

Since the somatoscope is such an expensive tool, at this point in time, there is no point reproducing it. The reason being that with our diachromic condenser, the research into somatidian theory can now continue without any possibility of it being lost because of lack of appropriate technology.

Question: Can you describe to us when you first saw somatids and what your feelings were—also do you remember the process that led to you discovering them?

Answer: I suspected something as a student when I looked at dry smears… What everyone called artefacts [i.e. something visible produced during the preparation of a slide which is not naturally present in the specimen] were always so perfectly reproduced.

After I graduated, and I was working with phase contrast microscopy on live-blood, I suspected they were some kind of 'particle'. At first, I thought they could be chylomicrons [a microscopic lipid particle common in the blood during fat digestion and assimilation].

But what they actually were became clear after the somatoscope had been built…

How? The large number of these shining particles was astonishing. This was a new challenge, a new perspective a new reality to better understand life… One thing was sure… if these particles were present in blood, they had to be there for one or more reasons. The body is so intelligent that no structure appears out of the blue or just for fun.

Question: You have written that somatids are 'eternal'—can you say a bit more about this?

Answer: Once somatids are in their resistant form, they appear to exist in nature eternally. However when proper environmental conditions become present, the resistant form returns to an active form again. We should note that somatids in blood are never in the resistant form.

After our death, all somatids return to their pleomorphic cycle thus turning the body into its basic mineral elements.

The somatids are needed to sustain life while alive (seemingly for purposes of cellular division and repair). They are needed after death to disintegrate the body, i.e. the decay process.

Question: What is it that causes the somatids to return to their three-stage cycle?

Answer: It is important to note that the somatids never return to their three-stage lifecycle. It is just as in life—in that we cannot go back to childhood.

Once the gate is crossed, the somatids continue their pleomorphic growth. However, if a change in the internal environment takes place—and the 'gate' gets put in place again—the somatids are once more limited to their three-stage cycle. 714-X helps achieve this—in that it influences the internal environmental of the body so that it is capable of sustaining life in harmony again.

Question: You often mention the phrase 'liquefying the lymph'—why doesn't the body do this itself?

Answer: When the body is being overcharged with toxins and metabolic waste, the lymph becomes thick and non-fluid. This is the terrain (le milieu) that sets the scene for degenerative diseases.

Question: Can we ask you to clarify the link between 714X, the somatids and cancer.

Answer: As you know, cancer is a disease where abnormal cellular division is occurring. Furthermore, abnormal cells are not detected soon enough by leucocytes (white blood cells). In a person dealing with cancer, leucocytes have lost their natural ability to detect abnormal cells before they reach a critical mass.

714X (by the design of its composition), is a product designed to give back to the white blood cells, (mostly neutrophiles, lymphocytes and monocytes), their original defence capacity towards foreign invasion (bacterial or viral). We can summarise the three concepts you raised in the question as follows (somatids—cancer —714X).

Somatids

Somatids are small live particles seen in the blood of all animals (and live plants). When proper biological balance is experienced by the body (i.e. a healthy state), somatids take the form of somatids, spores, double spores. This is the healthy range.

When a biological imbalance slowly progresses in the body (i.e. the gate control gets weaker and finally falls down), somatids are seen as advanced forms. That is from stage four to stage sixteen. Looking at the morphological patterns of somatids in live blood is an indirect way of measuring the state of the immune system. (Though of course, interpretation of the blood sample requires experience, skills in microscopy, and excellent comprehension of Somatidian Theory).

We should note that in a pre-cancerous condition, the full blown cycle is present (stages four to sixteen) and can be addressed before localisation of disease is confirmed through conventional biochemical blood tests.

714X and Cancer

What needs to be explained is the link between 714X and the cytokines. Since the mid-80's, but mostly since 1990, cytokines have been identified in the field of cellular biology—and are still today a very hot topic in the research world.

What are cytokines? Well, they are very small proteins found on the surface of white blood cells. They are crucially important in terms of immune system response.

A 1999 'in vitro' immune assay test performed with 714X, concluded that '714X appears to elevate the immune response and have some role in killing tumour cells'.[29]

Also, we now know *how* 714X works (in vitro) on the immune system. It appears that 714X mimics natural cytokines and therefore produces the same effect as these natural cytokines—but without the usual side effects of man made genetically engineered cytokines. Most likely it can mimic many cytokines but biochemical identification of new cytokines is not complete as it is still a very new and active field of research.

Before the immune assay test performed in 1999, we knew that 714X had a direct impact on leucocytes (white blood cells) via the observation of the mobility of cells under the microscope. At that time, all of our work, including the creation of 714X, was based on microscopic observations of the product on blood cells and somatidan forms. But since 1999, we have had the above mentioned biochemical proof. This brings strong evidence to support the claim that 714X works on the immune system.

We can summarise the above by saying that 714X is a restorative product for the full blown somatidian cycle. Specifically it restores the gate control and re-establishes the biological balance of blood back within a healthy range (visible on the microscope). On a cellular level, 714X mimics four different cytokines as follows:

- Tumour necrosis factor alpha (TNF-α)

- Interleukine 1 beta (IL-1β)

- Interleukine 6 (IL-6)

- Interleukine 8 (IL-8)

Because during cancer, the cytokines usually produced by white blood cells are no longer functioning properly, it makes it very easy for abnormal cells to multiply freely without any interference. 714X given in cancerous conditions can help the body to restore its normal defence mechanism by re-introducing cytokine activity.

714X helps to clean the body (lymphatic circulation is restored) and strongly supports the activity of cellular repair wherever damage is located (organ or system). 714X is not cytotoxic (cell killing). It does not kill cancerous cells but helps the body itself to eliminate these abnormal cells and restore normal immune functions.

Final Summary for this question:

In our view, cancer is not a local disease that tends to spread, but rather a general state of imbalance that eventually localises to the weakest organ and/or system. This conception of disease is quite different from conventional medicine.

714X is now better understood. Today, (in 2002), we know that the efficacy of 714X (biochemical wise) is related to its capacity to mimic cytokines as earlier discussed—and most important—is that it does this without any negative side-effects.

As we have always said, yes 714X can help; it can do 50% of the work in restoring health. But most important, the other 50% of the work to be done in recuperating from any degenerative disease has to be done by the person themselves. On this topic, it is our view that 'the mind-body connection' is crucial for healing. A few excellent references for this are: Dr. Bernie Seigel, Dr. Andrew Weil, Dr. Lorraine Day, Dr. Deepak Chopra, and Carolyn Myss.

Question: Have you trained individuals in somatidian science so work can continue in this on into the future?

Answer: Unfortunately there are very few people trained in the Naessens' blood test, though over the last five years we have trained some doctors, dentists, etc. However, though all of these people are very interested, few of them are true researchers. Also there is a lot of pressure on these people from the conventional establishment. So there is no great hope of continuation with these people and this is why we have stopped the trainings as we were giving them, and decided to invest in the future differently.

Instead we feel that the ideal situation is to train certified laboratory technicians in our blood test, as they already know how a microscope works. This will mean that screening clinics could be started in many different places (even mobile units if necessary) and could work to prevent degenerative disease. Ideally, doctors would know how to interpret the blood test, but laboratory technicians would perform it.

Cantron

Cantron is a product that was specifically formulated to help people heal from cancer. Recent laboratory tests recently carried out on Cantron confirm it possesses many remarkable qualities—and indicate that it is probably useful for people dealing with illness as well as for people interested in preventing cancer.

Cantron works in a variety of different ways upon the body. Summarised, they are as follows:

- Cantron targets cells that are functioning poorly because of damaged cellular respiration. Damaged cellular respiration means that a cells ability to generate energy by 'burning' carbohydrates in the presence of oxygen, has been permanently damaged and/or degraded. (Cancer cells have been documented to be cells with damaged respiration—more detail later.)

- Cantron acts as an extremely powerful antioxidant. Recent laboratory analysis has shown Cantron to be the most potent antioxidant known to mankind. (As we have discussed earlier in the book—see section on Boik's work p.34—antioxidants are considered to be important in dealing with free radicals. In terms of cancer, free radicals are thought to be a major factor underlying DNA damage. DNA damage in turn, is responsible for mutations of the cell that cause it to become cancerous.)

- Cantron functions as a chelating agent and detoxifier.

Cantron was developed by the late researcher and chemist James Sheridan (1912–2001). Sheridan described that he came up with the idea for Cantron after a series of related events. The events were as follows:

1   In 1931, while working in a laboratory with a group of professors and students, Sheridan witnessed a rare scientific phenomenon known as rhythmic banding. As a drop of a particular acid was added to a solution contained in a flask, the solution suddenly separated into six separate bands of colour—the colours of the rainbow in rainbow order: red, orange, yellow, green, blue and violet.

2   A month after the above experience, Sheridan began a three year project of reseach and study on the work of Professor Petrus Debye (a Dutch-born American physicist who won a 1936 Nobel Prize for his investigations on dipole movements and the diffraction of x-rays and electrons in gases.)

3 On the afternoon of September 6, 1936, while taking a nap, Sheridan had a dream in which his observation of the rhythmic banding phenomenon came together with his understanding of Deybe's work. This dream provided Sheridan with a great insight into the functioning of human cells and the inspiration needed to create Cantron.

Just how great an insight Sheridan gleaned can be gauged from the statement above, that Cantron is the most potent antioxidant known to mankind. Previously, the most powerful known antioxidants were OPC's (Oligomeric Proanthocyanidins), substances found in grape seeds and pine bark. ('OPC's are reported to be 20 times more effective than the vitamin C standard on water-soluble peroxyl radicals and 50 times more powerful than the vitamin E standard on fat-soluble peroxyl radicals'.[30])

A summary of the recent lab tests states that Cantron is:[31]

- Up to 1769 times more powerful than vitamin E on fat-soluble peroxyl radicals.

- Up to 424 times more powerful than vitamin C on water-soluble peroxyl radicals.

- Up to 45 times more powerful than Gallic acid on hydroxyl radicals

- Effective in blocking the formation of all superoxide radicals in the test system.

As well as being substantially more potent than vitamin E, C and Gallic acid, Cantron showed an ability to address more than one type of free radical (specifically, fat soluble and water soluble peroxyl radicals, superoxide radicals and hydroxyl radicals). Most often, a compound (e.g. vitamin C or E) is only active against one type of free radical. You can find a copy of the recent Cantron antioxidant study at www.healing-cancer.co.uk/resources

Sheridan's main aim with Cantron was to address the problem of damaged cellular respiration (defined as: the series of metabolic processes by which living cells produce energy through the oxidation of organic substances). Damaged cellular respiration has been shown to be a characteristic of cancer cells by various researchers. Please refer to Otto Warburg's Theory of Injured Cell Respiration, p.233 for more detailed information. Figure 2 illustrates the process that takes place within a cell (according to Sheridan) that causes it to become cancerous. Let's go through the process step-by-step, using Figure 2 for reference.

a) Cells are able to use various biochemical processes to generate energy. These various processes are represented on the diagram by the different levels (the various 'steps' on the 'ladder'). Biochemical processes used at the top of the ladder are able to generate more energy. Also, at each level the cell works at a different electrical potential—approximately 0.4 volts at the top of the ladder and 0.2v at the bottom.

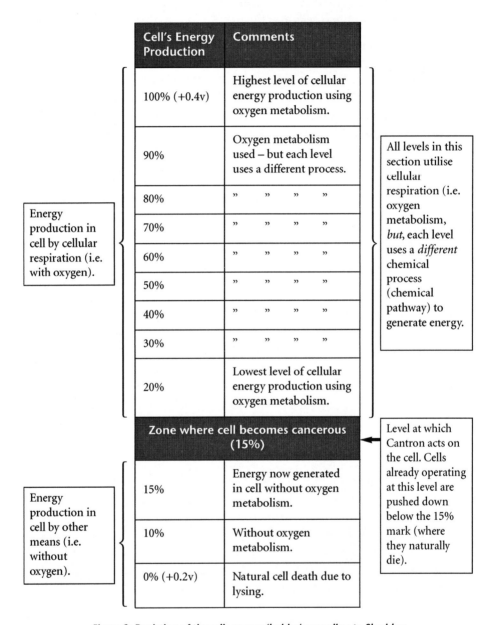

Figure 2: Depiction of the cells energy 'ladder' according to Sheridan

b) As described, though the cell can utilise different biochemical means of generating energy, we can group them into two main classes—with oxygen (aerobic) and without oxygen (anaerobic).

c) The shaded section (marked 'Zone where cell becomes cancerous') represents the point where the cell changes from energy production utilising oxygen (above the shaded zone), to energy production without oxygen (below the shaded zone). This changeover happens when the cell is operating at around 15 percent of its energy capability. Remember too, (even just above the 15 percent border zone mark) because each level in the cell uses different biochemical processes (even the different levels within the 'with oxygen metabolism' range), that the cell has stopped using the superior biochemical reactions that enable it to maintain its output close to 100 percent of capability, and is instead using inferior chemical processes.

d) If the cell manages to move into the zone below the shaded border zone, then it will not become cancerous. Below the zone, the cell will not be using oxygen to generate energy, but even so, the body will identify it as a damaged cell, and the cell will undergo lysis and die. (Lysis refers to the decomposition, dissolving and disintegration of a cell.)

e) Cells that remain in the border zone are the cells that become the problem cells—i.e. cancerous cells. While in the border zone they are neither one thing nor the other—they neither wholly use oxygen metabolism, nor its opposite, energy production through anaerobic biochemical processes. Further while they remain in the border zone the body is not able to identify them as problem cells and they will not be instructed to undergo lysis.

How Cantron Works

Cantron inhibits cellular respiration at a very specific level within the cell. In terms of Figure 2, the level Cantron works at, is at the level of the border zone. Therefore any cells already in the border zone will have their cellular respiration inhibited and will move downwards, into the area below the border zone. Though this will force them to start generating energy wholly without oxygen, the body will identify them as damaged cells and will instruct them to begin the process of lysis.

Question: What about cells higher up on the energy ladder (say operating at 80 percent), will they be affected and their energy output impaired by Cantron.

Answer: No. Remember, each level of the ladder uses a different chemical process—Cantron only affects the chemical process happening within the border zone (at around the 15 percent of energy output). Sheridan spent his lifetime finely tuning Cantron so that it would affect the process of cellular

Compound, (NCI's judgment)	Number of cell lines that showed mass reductions of at least:	
	80% reduction	90% reduction
Control—Perilly alcohol, (inactive)	0	0
Taxol, (active)	12	9
Cantron, (inactive)	32	18

Table 8: Mass reductions of Taxol & Cantron treated cell lines[35]

respiration within the border zone (and not the biochemical processes taking place higher up the ladder). Sheridan writes: 'Cantron's entire chemical structure was designed to inhibit respiration of cells at the critical point'.[32]

Reiterating the point written earlier, Cantron doesn't directly kill cells that have become cancerous (i.e. are operating in the border zone), rather by ensuring that such cells are pushed below the border zone the body's natural ability to instruct cells to die is called into play. Sheridan writes that Cantron will 'force the cancer cells further into the primitive stage where the body will attack and dispose of them naturally'.[33]

The National Cancer Institute (NCI) Cantron Test

By 1990/1 there was such an interest in Cantron that the NCI agreed to conduct a small study into its functioning. The study was quite straightforward; Cantron and a leading chemotherapeutic agent (Taxol) were compared in their effectiveness against sixty types of cancer cell. The study was carried out 'in-vitro', i.e. outside the body in test tubes, over a period of two days.

For each type of cancer cell the NCI study measured two factors:

1   The kill rate of each agent.

2   The change in mass (weight) of the various cancer cell cultures in response to each agent.

We should also be aware that Taxol (the chemotherapeutic agent used) is considered the gold standard of chemotherapy. Even so, Taxol is a toxic agent and can produce many undesirable side effects in individuals who use it.

The results of the NCI study

In terms of the kill rate of cancer cells for each compound, Taxol was clearly superior to Cantron. The official conclusion of the study draws heavily on this finding. In part it reads:

> 'It should also be noted that [Cantron] was completely devoid of cancer cell-killing activity in 37% of the cell lines tested…'[34]

Bearing in mind that Cantron is completely non-toxic, especially in comparison with Taxol, it seems strange that the above statement is in the negative. Instead, it might have stated that Cantron had a cell killing effect in 63 percent of cell lines—and quantified exactly how Cantron's kill rate compared with Taxol's. However, possibly the most important finding of the study isn't mentioned in the official conclusion. The data reveals that Cantron had a significant effect on cell mass for many of the cancel cell lines. Here is a table that compares the change in mass for cell lines treated with Taxol and with Cantron.

You can see that if we consider mass reductions of eighty percent, then twelve types of cancer cells experienced this reduction of mass when treated with Taxol compared with 32 types with Cantron. If we consider a ninety percent reduction (obviously a very significant reduction in mass), then nine types of

Brand name	Comments
Entelev	Original formulation by James Sheridan
Cantron	A further development of Entelev as directed by Sheridan
Cancell/Dark Cancell	Similar formulation to Entelev/Cantron produced by Ed Sopcak (a scientist who worked as part of the original Cantron production team)
Clear Cancell/ Quantrol	A supposed 'chemical free' or 'homeopathic' version of Dark Cancell produced by Ed Sopcak. Bears no resemblance to Entelev/Cantron as formulated by James Sheridan.
Protocel	A version that appeared in 2000 based on the original Entelev formula and produced by a Canadian company (Remission and Wellness) working in conjunction with the Sheridan family. Considered to be a good product.
New Millenium Cantron	A further development of the original Cantron and the one used in the recent laboratory antioxidant tests.

Table 9: Clarification Of Product Brand Names

cancer cells experienced this level of reduction in mass when treated with Taxol, compared to eighteen types when treated with Cantron.

You can find more detailed results data (upon which the above table is based) in Appendix G: NCI Cantron Test Data. We are sure you will agree with us, that the above described mass reductions would seem to be extremely significant, and at least worth a mention. Proponents of Cantron, assert that mass reduction, and not direct cancer cell kills, is what is to be expected from Cantron—as it pushes cells in the border zone, down below the border zone, to a place where they will be naturally instructed by the body to die (lysis). It is claimed that lysis and the consequent dying of cancer cells is a lengthy process taking months rather than days and that if the study had been run for a much longer period than two days then the mass reductions would have eventually translated into cancer cell deaths.

We take the position that the mass reductions found in the NCI study do not necessarily indicate that Cantron heals cancer in the body. As described, this was an in-vitro test rather than a human study and in-vitro studies do not necessarily translate to the same effects in human beings. However, the results are very promising and do seem to fit in with Sheridan's model of how Cantron seeks to act on cancer cells, and it would seem sensible for the NCI and/or other governmental bodies to investigate the compound further, especially in light of the recent findings about Cantron's antioxidant ability.

How to take Cantron

¼ teaspoon (1.25cc) of Cantron should be taken every four to six hours, with the last dose before bedtime made up to ½ a teaspoon (2.5cc). Maintaining a constant level of Cantron is more important than increasing the dose. Cantron can be taken mixed with water or juice and is best drunk on an empty stomach.

Several other supplements have been observed to interfere with Cantron's functioning, and it is therefore recommended these not be taken during the period in which Cantron is being used. The most important substances to avoid are Coenzyme Q10, high doses of vitamins C, E and the mineral selenium.

Full instructions for using Cantron are available from the manufacturer, Medical Research Products (Florida).

In recent toxicity tests Cantron has been shown to be twenty times safer than aspirin and animal experiments have shown no side effects even when seven hundred times the recommended dose was injected into the body cavities of mice.

Clarification of product names

Since James Sheridan began synthesising Entelev soon after its conception in 1936, it has been known by a variety of names. In addition some other individuals/companies produced their own versions and marketed them under their own brand names. In terms of a reliable and documented product we recommend New Millennium Cantron manufactured by Medical Research Products of Florida. Medical Research Products worked extensively with Sheridan refining and improving the formula. Protocel by Renewal & Wellness is also closely based on Sheridan's original Entelev and is considered to be a well produced formula.

Price of New Millennium Cantron

New Millennium Cantron (8 fl oz) 3-week supply costs: $60 (£33)

New Millennium Cantron (32 fl oz) 4-month supply costs: $190 (£105)

Supplier

Medical Research Products
3960 NW 167 Street
Miami, FL USA
33054

Web: www.medresproducts.com
Email: gpg911@cantron.com
☎: (001) 305-628-0981
📠: (001) 305-628-2091

Price of Protocel

Protocel comes in two variants: Formula 23 & Formula 50. Formula 50 is the most recent variant of the formulation.

Protocel Formula 23 (16 fl oz) 2-month supply: $98.00 (£54)
Protocel Formula 23 (2 x 16 fl oz) 4-month supply: $180.00 (£100)

Protocel Formula 50 (16 fl oz) 2½ month supply: $130.00 (£72)
Protocel Formula 50 (2 x 16 fl oz) 5 month supply: $242.00 (£134)

Supplier

Renewal & Wellness
110 South Main Street
Simpsonville
SC 29681
☎: (001) 864 962 8880
Web: www.protocel.com

B-17 and Hydrazine Sulphate

In the following two sections we will take a look at two remaining compounds that deserve a mention. The first, B-17, is worthy of discussion because it has been used by tens of thousands of individuals (many of whom have claimed it was a useful treatment)—and because it is employed in many alternative cancer clinics as a complementary treatment. However we should note that though many reliable medical doctors attest to the value of B-17 as a cancer therapy, human studies demonstrating benefit have not yet been carried out (see section starting p.243 for results of animal studies).

The second compound we shall discuss is Hydrazine Sulphate, an easily available, relatively non-toxic chemical used for the refining of rare metals, an antioxidant in solder flux and many other industrial processes. Hydrazine Sulphate is an interesting compound that has shown (in various trials) to help with cachexia (severe weight loss) in individuals dealing with late stage cancer. We shall look at some of the results from these studies.

B-17

B-17 (otherwise known as laetrile or amygdalin) is a substance that can act directly against cancer cells. This is because it contains a molecule of cyanide that, though normally safely locked up, can be released by enzymes present in cancer cells. Thus B-17 can deliver targeted, lethal dosages of cyanide molecules, exactly where they are needed most (i.e. right next to cancer cells). You can read full details of its operation in the section entitled The B-17 (p.243).

First however, we should point out that if you know of a medical doctor who can carry out intravenous infusion of B-17 then this may be your best choice. He will be able to combine the B-17 with other substances such as vitamins to increase the overall effect. In fact it is always recommended that B-17 be taken along with a comprehensive range of enzymes and vitamins so that the B-17 forms just one part of a multifaceted approach to cancer.

The simplest choice open to you is to take amygdalin tablets. It is recommended that you work up to 3000mg per day (2 × 500mg / three times a day). The amygdalin tablets should be taken on an empty stomach—along with a full glass of water—and the last set of tablets should be taken just before bedtime.

The dose should be built up slowly over a number of days (starting with just 500mg per day) to ensure that there is no allergic, or other type reaction. Reactions are very rare—though if one does happen then you will need to stop taking the amygdalin, and consult with your health practitioner. Possible reactions could include rapid heartbeat, shortness of breath, muscle weakness, light-headedness, dizziness and nausea. (Usually, if this happens, your health practitioner will suggest you have a break for a few days and then re-introduce the amygdalin at a lower dose).

For supply of all the above amygdalin products contact CytoPharma de Mexico: www.cytopharma.com

Cost of 100% pure amygdalin tablets:

Bottle with one hundred tablets 500mg – £49.40 ($79)
This works out approx. £88.75 ($142) per month

Cost of intravenous therapy:

It is difficult to give definitive costs for intravenous amygdalin. In the US each infusion is likely to cost $100–$200 and in the UK around the £90–£100 mark—though the exact cost will depend upon other substances included in the infusion. As you can appreciate, the costs of the therapy can soon add up. (It is not so much the raw materials, rather physician time and skill).

It is suggested that infusions are carried out daily in three cycles of twelve injections—though each physician is likely to have their own favoured protocol.

It is also possible to take amygdalin in the form of apricot kernels—as these do contain appreciable amounts. However, because apricot kernels do not come in standardised dosages and are difficult to take in large quantity's, we recommend that you use the tablet form of B-17. However, in terms of preventative health, we should note that Krebs (one of B-17's main proponents) recommends ten kernels a day for life. An internet search will bring up a list of Apricot kernel suppliers such as: www.ourfathersfarm.com

As already mentioned, amygdalin should always be used in conjunction with other cancer therapies. The most important of these are considered to be enzyme and vitamin supplementation.

Please see the detailed section on enzyme supplementation starting on p.78 as to the type of enzymes required and how they should be taken.

Other compounds regularly combined with amygdalin:

- Vitamin E – water soluble form
- Vitamin C – to bowel tolerance limit (see p.222)

- Emulsified (water-based) Beta Carotene – 30,000 I.U. per day – three times a day after meals.

- Emulsified (water-based) vitamin A – 125,000 I.U.

In addition, take the beta-carotene and vitamin A at different times of the day and ensure they are water-based forms—high dosages of 'oil only' forms can lead to liver toxicity and damage.

(Note: You should only take above dosages of emulsified beta-carotene/ vitamin A under medical supervision).

Cost of therapy: See discussion above for details.

Where to obtain it: See links above for suppliers of amygdalin.

The therapy is available intravenously in the UK at Munro-Hall Clinic (www.hallvtox.dircon.co.uk).

Some US providers of intravenous B-17 can be found listed on this page: www.whale.to/cancer/laetrile.html

And an international listing can be found on this page:

www.cancure.org/laetrile.htm

Hydrazine Sulphate

Theoretical Underpinnings: Hydrazine sulphate, or Sehydrin as it is known in Russia, has shown itself to be an extremely valuable therapeutic agent—especially for individuals experiencing cachexia (severe weight loss). It has shown particularly good results against brain cancers, which traditionally are some of the most difficult cancers to treat.

Several well-run clinical trials have shown hydrazine sulphate to produce subjective responses in around 50–70% of patients and objective response rates around the 20% mark. Subjective responses refer to improvements such as an increase in appetite, cessation of weight loss and/or weight gain, and a decrease in pain. Objective responses refer to measurable reductions in tumour size and a decrease in cancer-associated complications such as jaundice.

Side effects experienced by patients are rare, and generally mild in nature, e.g. dizziness, tiredness or slight numbness in fingers and toes (occasionally nausea is reported). Interestingly, during various trials it has been noted that hydrazine sulphate significantly lifts the mood of individuals taking it.

Within the conventional cancer field, subjective responses are often considered the poor cousin to objective responses. Ironically, however, it is not cancer that is directly responsible for most deaths, but cachexia—the wasting away of an individual as their cancer tumour demands more and more of the available nutrients. It is estimated that cachexia is the condition that underlies 77% of cancer patient deaths.

In the late 1960's, Dr. Joseph Gold came up with an idea. Instead of focussing on killing cancer cells via direct methods such as chemotherapy or radiation, why not focus instead on preventing the actual cause of death in most cases—cachexia. Moreover, he suggested that preventing cachexia might itself feed back and cause a regression, or slowing down, of tumour growth.

The process in the body that causes cachexia in cancer patients has been known for a long time. Cancer cells require large amounts of glucose—which in turn, they convert to lactic acid. Also, because cancer cells are not as efficient as normal body cells, it is estimated that they consume over ten times as much glucose. Moreover, they only partly metabolise the glucose and it is returned back into the body as lactic acid.

The body, via the liver, is able to recycle this lactic acid back into glucose via an enzymic process known as gluconeogenesis. It is this natural process that cancer cells take so much advantage of. Though at first it is in the background, and not particularly noticeable, over time, cancer cells requisition more and more of an individuals liver capacity for the process of gluconeogenesis—leaving less and less liver capacity to service other metabolic requirements.

It is this process that usually leads to the complete wasting of the cancer patient's body. Further, even with comprehensive nutritional therapy, cachexia is seldom preventable.

Dr Gold suggested that if this process of gluconeogenesis could be interrupted, then it might well have a profound impact upon the patient's health and well-being. He characterised the relationship between cancer and an individual's liver as a 'sick relationship', and suggested that interrupting and breaking this relationship will starve tumours of their primary fuel source, and enable the liver to once again work for the benefit of the whole body. A short while after publishing this hypothesis, Dr. Gold came across exactly the type of agent he had been looking for—hydrazine sulphate. In 1975 he conducted the first human trial using the substance.

Since then numerous studies have been carried out—the majority of them producing results similar to those mentioned above. However, Dr. Gold has hit a 'brick wall' in the western world with regard to hydrazine's acceptance by conventional medical authorities. Much more interest and use of hydrazine sulphate has been made in Russia, and several large scale clinical trials have been carried out. The abstract of a 1994 study concerning the impact of hydrazine sulphates on patients dealing with brain cancer reads:

> 'The results of Sehydrin administration in forty-six patients with malignant and six patients with benign tumours of the brain are presented. Pronounced therapeutic effect for the whole group was 63.5% and 73%, if partial regression of neurological symptoms in the entire brain and separate foci is considered. The percentages for patients with malignant tumours only were 61 and 71.1, respectively.
>
> Since Sehydrin has virtually no significant untoward side effects, it is considered a most safe medication for the management of brain tumours. It is recommended in cases of inoperable tumour and for post-operative adjuvant chemotherapy with a view toward extending the patient's survival time and improving the quality of life.'[36]

A question often asked is: if the blocking of the enzyme responsible for gluconeogenesis of lactic acid causes other problems in the body, i.e. surely if gluconeogenesis of lactic acid is a necessary part of body functioning, then aren't other problems likely to appear if its functioning is blocked? The answer to this lies in the fact that cancer cells are not as sophisticated as the body itself. Though cancer cells need to use this pathway for recycling lactic acid back into glucose, the body has other similar chemical pathways it can use for its own purposes. (You may remember John Boik's answer to a similar question about signalling pathways within cells—see interview with Boik p.34)

As mentioned, hydrazine sulphate is a low cost compound and there is every reason to employ it as a therapy—especially if you are experiencing cachexia. It is important the hydrazine sulphate is of reagent-equivalent grade (i.e. 100% pure), as an impure version is often used for industrial purposes.

Incorporating Hydrazine Sulphate therapy is very straightforward. You will need to obtain some hydrazine sulphate from a reputable supplier. A search on an Internet search engine will bring up plenty of overseas suppliers.

It is generally recommended that you take hydrazine sulphate according to the following schedule (hydrazine sulphate usually comes in 60-mg capsules, and these should be taken one to two hours before meals):

- You should begin with one 60mg capsule a day for three days.

- If you feel your response is good (i.e. you do not have any reactions) you should take two 60mg capsules a day for three days.

- Again if you feel that your response is good, you can increase the dosage further to three 60mg capsules a day for three days.

- If after taking three 60mg capsules a day for three days your response is still good, then you should stay on this dosage (as long as you do not have any reactions). If three times a day is too much, you should reduce it back down to two 60mg capsules a day again.

Note: Three days either side of taking hydrazine sulphate, it is recommended that you should consume NO sedatives, tranquillisers, barbiturates, alcohol of any kind, anti-depressants, vitamin B-6, or over-the-counter cold and allergy remedies.

Also, foods high in tyramine should be avoided as hydrazine sulphate acts as a monoamine oxidase (MAO) inhibitor (an enzyme in the body responsible for breaking down certain neurotransmitters).

These include:

- Smoked, pickled, fermented and similarly processed meats

- Foods containing aged cheeses

- Fish and soy products

- Fava beans and ripe figs

- Chianti and other red wines

- Foods containing monosodium glutamate (MSG)

See the article on the Kathy Keeton Foundation page entitled 'Diet Do's and Dont's' for a more detailed list of food to avoid. On this site you will also find a few other articles about hydrazine sulphate from notable doctors and researchers. You will find the site at:

www.kathykeeton-cancer.org

Cost: You should aim to work slowly up to three × 60mg tablets as described above. The cost of taking three × 60mg capsules a day is around £27.50 ($44) per month.

How to order: We list two suppliers:

Medical Research Products
3960 NW 167 Street
Miami, FL USA
33054

Web: www.medresproducts.com
Email: gpg911@cantron.com
☎: (001) 305-628-0981
🖷: (001) 305-628-2091

Also available from:

http://life.uniserve.com/expl/hydrazin.htm
ben@uniserve.com

5

Group 3 Therapies – Clinic Based Cancer Therapies

G ROUP 3 THERAPIES represent some of your most important choices. These are the therapies that have proved themselves, or are in the process of proving themselves, to be some of the most effective non-toxic cancer therapies around. Therapies in this group have been listed separately because they require you to visit a particular clinic—at least to begin the therapy. They will also cost you considerably more than the other therapies. However, the costs are not prohibitive—in most cases they represent the cost of an average family car—and in some cases substantially less. For instance, Dr Lechin's therapy will only cost you a few thousand pounds.

Important note: There is a chance, that by the time you read this book, Dr Lechin's therapy will have become available in Europe and the US—as well as being available for a lower cost. Please check the following URL to find the current availability and pricing:

www.healing-cancer.co.uk

It is important we address the common fear, about the individuals who run these sort of clinics, as they are often seen as quacks, predators or as selfish, greedy or unscrupulous individuals. We would like to assure you that you are not going to be 'ripped off' by any of the clinics we will list. Rather, for what you will receive, they represent very good value for money. All the clinics use very specialised equipment, synthesise very specialised compounds and employ doctors and health professionals. Also, in contrast to conventional cancer hospitals and facilities, none of these clinics receive any funding or help—they have to meet the whole cost of providing their services from patient fees. As a comparison, the bill for a week's stay in a UK hospital for a straightforward operation (e.g. hip replacement) comes to around £8,000 ($12,800)—and this is a subsidised figure. Please note: though some cancer clinics in Mexico are regarded as centres of excellence, this does not apply to all of them. For an excellent description of a checkout visit to several Mexican Clinics see Penelope Williams account in Alternatives in Cancer Therapy (Key Porter Books:2000).

For each therapy, we shall take a look at its theoretical base—and then present an interview with either its founder, or other prime authority on the therapy. This is so that you can hear about the therapies first-hand, from doctors who are experienced at working with them day in and day out.

Dr Lechin's Neuroimmunomodulation Approach to Cancer

Dr Lechin's Neuroimmunomodulation Approach to Cancer involves therapeutically manipulating neurotransmitters in the brain so as to directly affect the functioning of the immune system. It shows extremely promising results, is non-toxic and can proceed in conjunction with other non-toxic anti-cancer therapies. Furthermore, it is based on solid science and research, including the neurochemical profiling and treatment of over twenty-five thousand individuals dealing with a variety of illnesses and diseases. Dr Lechin, a Venezuelan doctor and researcher, has pioneered this technique over the last thirty years. As of writing, he is seventy-five years of age, still running a busy clinical practice and carrying out associated research. Dr Lechin's Neuroimmunomodulation Approach to Cancer (as well as other somatic and psychological illnesses) represents the culmination of his life's work.

Dr Lechin has documented (along with complete clinical records including X-ray evidence) many instances of recovery from cancer, using neuroimmunomodulation techniques. However, though Dr Lechin has published over one hundred and seventy research papers detailing aspects of his approach, in common with other 'cutting edge' researchers, he has found it difficult to find wider acceptance of his findings and associated therapy. He writes:

> 'Up to the present we have treated some three thousand advanced cancer patients. Most came to our institute when all conventional therapies had failed. We have presented our results in the most important cancer hospitals of the US...

> ...It is not our intention to announce a cure for malignant diseases, but to demonstrate the close association existing between uncoping stress situation, Th-2 immune profile, and malignant disease. When we lectured, by invitation at conferences in several US oncology hospitals and universities, oncologists were greatly impressed. However they asked us for a package treatment like chemotherapy and radiotherapy. They could not accept treatments based on neuropharmacological, neuroendocrinal or neuroimmunilogical manipulations. Their hospitals are not provided with neurochemical laboratories. These specialists felt unable to design appropriate neuropharmacological therapy according to neurochemical + immunological findings. Unfortunately this obstacle is still present. For our part, we continued applying our therapeutical approach on cancer patients attending our institute and gave up reporting our

experience to medical journals because they lacked adequate reviewers and asked for double blind studies...'[37]

Seventy-five of Dr Lechins published papers detailing the approach with a variety of conditions are stored in the PubMed database. You can access abstracts of these studies by following the following instructions.

First go to the home page of the National Center for Biotechnology Information at: www.ncbi.nih.gov and enter 'Lechin F.' as the search text. Then change the 'what-to-search' drop down box so it reads 'PubMed', and click 'Go'. The titles of relevant study will be brought up on screen. If you wish to read the associated abstracts, you can change the drop down box next to the 'Display' button to 'Abstract'—and then click the 'Display' button.

A more complete listing of Dr Lechin's studies (over 145 of them), as well as books detailing the approach can be found at:

www.lechin.com/refeframe.htm

Dr Lechin is working hard at communicating his findings to clinical doctors around the world so they can begin using this promising and revolutionary approach to illness. To this end, he has recently published a book detailing both the theoretical foundations of the neuroimmunomodulation approach to illness as well as detailing how doctors can implement it as a therapy for their patients. It is a detailed and technical book, specifically aimed at the practicing physician and is titled Neurocircuitry and Neuroautonomic Disorders: Reviews and Therapeutic Strategies (published by Karger).

The basis of Dr Lechin's approach is a profiling of an individual's main neurotransmitters, particularly in terms of the ratios they are present in relation to each other. Neurotransmitters are chemicals secreted by various parts of the brain and are responsible for the functioning of parts of the body such as the immune system and the endocrine system.

The main neurotransmitters profiled by Dr Lechin are noradrenaline, adrenaline, dopamine, free serotonin, total seratonin, and tryptophane. The profile usually includes other immune and biological markers measured through standard blood tests. (It is important to note the above neurotransmitter profiling is carried out using blood serum measurements—not urine type measurements as are more commonly available).

An individual's neurotransmitters are measured at various times during a challenge test, i.e. an individual is given a substance (e.g. busispone) that causes a change in neurotransmitter levels for a couple of hours. Neurotransmitter levels are measured at various times during the challenge test, and then plotted on a graph. When analysed, the results provide in-depth information about how an individual's immune system is functioning. Further, an individual's profile can be compared with known profiles of both health and illness.

For instance the ratio of Noradrenaline to adrenaline has been found to be very significant. From the thousands of profiles carried out, it has been established that when the ratio is low (e.g. less than 2:1), it usually indicates an individual is badly adjusted (physiologically) to stress's in their life. Dr Lechin has named a profile such as this, 'uncoping stress profile'. It should, however, be borne in mind that the reading of challenge test results in conjunction with all the other measurements takes significant skill and expertise. Dr Lechin would therefore like to see an increase in relevant training for doctors so that they can interpret and understand neuropharmaceutical data. His view is that only then will we be able to use neuropharmaceutical agents in a beneficial and individually tailored way. In contrast, at the present time, for illnesses for which such drugs are employed (e.g. mental health issues), they are administered in a 'one size fits all' manner—specified by drug manufacturers.

The actual therapy focuses on 'nudging' a patient's neurological profile towards one that is found in healthy individuals. The particular benefit for cancer patients (usually Th2 profile—apart from Hodgkin's lymphoma and pancreatic adenocarcinoma) of pushing their profile towards a healthy state includes enhanced cellular immunity. That is, as their profile is normalised, they will likely show increased activity of their immune system—for example, increased killer cell activity, which in turn is beneficial in terms of the body being able to deal with tumours and rogue cancer cells that might metastasise.

A typical therapy for a Th2 profiled patient might include some or all of the following (it is worth noting that Dr Lechin only uses very low doses of the following medicines and that they need to be taken at fairly precise times of the day):

1 NA (Noradrenaline) precursors (L-tyrosine, L-phenylalanine)

2 NA-releasing agents

3 Small doses of β-blocking agents

4 NA uptake inhibitors

5 NA + dopamine enhancer drug

6 Small dosages of 5HT precursor before bed

The impact of the medications are monitored closely and adjusted as needed. After a period of time, an individual should be re-profiled to check how their neurochemical profile has altered in response to therapy. As discussed above, the experience of Dr Lechin and his team has shown that as an individual's profile normalises so they move towards a state of normal health.

Dr Lechin has published several studies on his work with cancer patients. In a 1987 paper Dr Lechin presented visual evidence from twenty-two representative cases—demonstrating how tumours had responded to therapeutic medication provided. (All patients stopped other cancer therapies before beginning Dr Lechin's protocol). A similar 1989 paper also providing photographic evidence of the improvements of individuals on the therapy is equally impressive.

Another paper entitled 'Successful Immunopharmacological Therapy of thirty-seven Metastatic Cancer Patients' reports:

> 'All patients improved significantly, with improvement rated as follows:
>
> 1   Total remission of tumour and metastases (nine cases)
>
> 2   Significant (50%) reduction of metastases and survival up to the present time (thirteen cases)
>
> 3   Halt in metastases progression plus survival up to the present (seven cases)
>
> 4   Slowing of metastases progression plus three-fold increase of life expectancy (eight cases)
>
> All patients, including those of Group IV, remained symptom less throughout treatment…'

It is worth noting that Dr Lechin has applied the above therapeutic principles to many other illnesses with successful results including myasthenia, thrombocytopenic pupura, Guillain-Barre, bipolar syndrome, rheumatoid arthritis, multiple sclerosis, Crohn's enteritis and others. In our view, treating illness by modifying an individual's neurotransmitter profile is an approach to health and disease that will 'burst' onto the global stage over the next 10–20 years. It is an approach that has enormous potential because the neurotransmitters are the 'puppet strings' that control and coordinate all of the systems in the body.

Clinic Details:

If you wish to call, the clinic is open in the mornings (until 13-00)—however not all the clinic staff speak English and so you might do better sending a fax.

☎:   (582) 574 2568   or (582) 574 2702   or (582) 574 4819
         (582) 574 9953   or (582) 574 2702   or (582) 574 8842

📠:   (582) 575 3161   or (582) 961 0172

Email: flechin@telcel.net.ve

Web: www.lechin.com

Address: Dr Fuad Lechin
Av, Panteon – Piso 8 – 805 – 807 y 812
Anexo al Hospital de Clinicas Caracas
San Bernardino
Caracas
Venezuela

Cost of therapy: Blood tests and initial medication to take home approx £2000- £3333 (3000-5000 US dollar).

Above cost does not include accommodation—but the clinic can help you arrange this. A room in a nearby hotel with three meals a day costs around £41.88 ($67) per day.

How to go about receiving the therapy: The therapy is very easy to carry out at home once you have had the appropriate blood tests carried out. At present there are only a few laboratories in the world that are able to carry out the blood serum tests needed—and the only one available for public use is Dr Lechin's clinic in Caracus, Venezuela. Dr Lechin's clinic is sited in the brand new Clinic de Caracas, a newly constructed hospital near the centre of the city.

The relevant blood tests (to establish your present immune system profile) can be carried out the day after you arrive. The results take three or four days to come back. Dr Lechin's team will then prescribe appropriate medication to move your immune profile back towards one that represents full health. You will need to stay around the clinic for a couple of weeks while Dr Lechin's team assess the impact of your medication.

Once Dr Lechin's team feel confident that your medication is moving your immune profile in the right direction, you can return home. Once home, you continue taking the prescribed medication—though long term, you will need to source this from your local doctor or other health professional.

It is best to return to the clinic at a future date (e.g. six months) to have a repeat profiling carried out. This will establish the exact impact of the medication upon the various systems of your body. Additional fine-tuning will be carried out if necessary.

Availability of Dr Lechin's therapy in Europe & the US

As already mentioned in the introduction to Group 3 Therapies—there is a good chance that the therapy (including the relevant neurochemical profiling) has become available in the Europe & the US. Please check the following URL for up-to-date information:

www.healing-cancer.co.uk/resources

Q And A With Dr Lechin (Neuroimmunomodulation)

Simon Kelly: Can you begin by describing the number of individuals with cancer you have treated—how successful you feel you have been, and how you treat cancer.

Dr Fuad Lechin: We have successfully treated around three thousand cancer patients. We have obtained very high success with stomach, prostate, ovarian and kidney cancer patients.

And we have successfully treated hundreds of advanced breast cancers. However, we also prescribed surgery before or after our therapeutic manipulations.

Our therapeutic approach is based on neuropharmacological manipulations. These are addressed so as to enhance a person's immunological activity. In my opinion, neuroimmunomodulation is the best available procedure to trigger macrophage activity [a type of white blood cell which can kill cancer cells]. These cells are responsible for the release of the cytokines—IL2, IL12, IL18, and interferon, TNF etc [all important substances released by the body in its fight against cancer].

We have correlated that cancer, stress and the immune system are very intertwined. Cancer can disappear and reappear—according to stressful events.

SK: Can you explain about the immune profiling procedure. If an individual is to find a laboratory that can carry out the appropriate blood profiling for them, what are the minimum tests that they need to have done?

FL: They need to have a neurochemical profile carried out—i.e. the levels of plasma neurotransmitters (in blood) such as noradrenaline, adrenaline, dopamine, free serotonin, total seratonin, and tryptophan.

SK: Should the neurotransmitters be measured during a challenge test (stress test) or can they just have a snapshot of their neurochemical profile carried out after fasting for a number of hours?

FL: It should be during a challenge test—there are several possible stress tests that we use. For instance:

- Orthostasis [i.e. standing upright] and exercise

- Oral glucose challenge

- Burpirone challenge

There are some others—we can advise on the most suitable type of stress test.

SK: What about if a person can't locate a lab to do their neurochemical profile—is it possible to send you a sample of blood for testing here in Venezuela?

FL: I am afraid it is not possible to do this.

SK: Let's suppose someone comes to you for the blood test and then returns home to begin initial treatment. Are you and your team able to support patients and their doctors from a distance—have you worked like this before?

FL: Yes it is perfectly possible—and yes we have done it before.

SK: Let's say a person dealing with cancer preferred to stay in Venezuela to receive treatment. What time period would they need to stay for you to really tailor the therapy for them, and for them to see a difference? In addition, what sort of cost would they be looking at?

FL: I would say that their length of stay would need to be around two to three months—and the cost of this treatment (excluding accommodation and food), would be around 3,000 – 5,000 US dollars.

SK: Do patients ever experience any serious side effects from the drug treatment that you prescribe.

FL: Never. No undesirable side effects occur—on the contrary, only desirable side effects.

SK: What about surgery for cancer patients—what are your recommendations regarding this?

FL: Surgery is necessary, usually in all cases. It removes a high number of malignant cells and thus facilitates the neuro-immunological therapy.

SK: Can you explain why you include recommendations for small amounts of both levamisole and methotrexate (chemotherapy agents) in your prescriptions for some patients? I was surprised to see the mention of the use of these agents in your protocol. What is your feeling about chemotherapy in general?

FL: Well levamisole enhances Th1 activity. It is useful from this perspective [when used in very small amounts].

Chemotherapy is addressed to kill malignant cells. However, macrophages are destroyed by chemotherapeutical agents as well. These agents tend to kill macrophages before they eliminate all malignant cells.

I should point out that we can only treat previously non-treated cancer patients. Experience has taught us we cannot help patients who have received chemotherapy and/or radiotherapy. There are only two types of cancer patients who should be treated with those therapies: Hodgkin's lymphoma and testes cancer.

SK: You have mentioned Th-1 and Th-2 immune profiles—can you say what these correspond to?

FL: Humoral immunty = Th2 immunity. This is the side of the immune system that is most linked with antibody production.

Cellular immunity = Th1 immunity. This is the side of the immune system most linked with cellular immunity—e.g. macrophages. This is the side of the immune system that it is usually important to stimulate in the cancer patient.

Although we have successfully treated many hundreds of cancer patients, our major concern is with the neuropharmacological therapeutic approach to almost all diseases. Drugs which act at central nervous system level trigger changes at the immune system. It is called neuroim-munomodulation.

There are two types of diseases: Th-1 predominant and Th-2 predominant diseases. Neuroimmunomodulation is addressed to find Th1 = Th2 balance. For instance, bronchial asthma, myasthenia gravis, gastroduo-denal ulcer, infectious diseases, parasitic diseases and most types of cancer are included amongst Th-2 predominant diseases. Conversely, multiple sclerosis, rheumathic diseases, Crohn's diseases etc. are included into Th-1 predominant diseases. There are other diseases which show oscillations between these two poles. (Systemic Lupus is the typical example of the latter group).

SK: In your work you stress the importance of sleep—in terms of the correct regulation of neurotransmitters. You point out that the different stages of sleep are vitally important in enabling us maintaining a strong immune system. In connection with this, how come some people (e.g. Mrs Thatcher) are reputed to be able to get by with only a few hours of sleep a night?

Further, what about people who work odd shift hours—what is your recommendation to them?

FL: It is my opinion that Mrs Thatcher became old quite prematurely. I think this happened because she is a poor sleeper. A person can sleep during the day or the night. However, you should sleep enough and deeply enough.

In terms of the stages of sleep, there are two important stages: slow wave associated sleep and REM associated sleep. REM sleep is necessary for memory consolidation while slow wave sleep is necessary for things like somatic restoration, immunity, anti-stress etc.

SK: How practical is it for clinical doctors to learn enough about neurochemistry required to carry out your therapy. A few pages from your last book might send many doctors running for cover. It seems to require a very detailed understanding of neurochemistry. Without this understanding, patients will end up being treated with standard dosages and treatments.

FL: This is absolutely true. It took me forty years to build the bridge between basic science and medicine—you should remember that I am an MD, a psychoanalyst, a physiologist, a pharmacologist and a mathematician as well as possessing a great deal of immunological information.

For the above reasons, I am a lonely man. I feel that most doctors do not understand what I explain. In addition, the history of medical science tends not to be written in small countries, like Venezuela—rather at the present time, truth is the private property of the USA (just as the UK was the owner of 'truth' for the last three hundred years).

SK: Bearing this in mind (i.e. that very few doctors possess the skill and understanding necessary to use medications to accurately manipulate neurochemicals in the brain), would it really be that bad if people were treated with standard regimes and dosages—i.e. doctors could give cancer patients a typical drug prescription and see whether it works?

FL: I am afraid that this simplistic approach does not work. It is necessary to manipulate many variables in order to reach the target. Doctors should be aware about the physiological disorders underlying the symptoms. It is a new language that should be understood by doctors.

SK: What about critics of unconventional cancer therapies such as Saul Green, who maintain that there is no immune surveillance over cancer? He would claim, for instance, that the immune system of most cancer patients is indicated to be perfectly normal if tests are carried out.

FL: It is very difficult to state that the immune system of cancer patients is normal. Today we know that there are many, many variables that need to be investigated in order to establish the concept of 'normality' of the immune system. Saul Green is an ignorant man about this issue.

SK: What about food—what role can foods play in your system—i.e. do you see your treatment supported and enhanced by particular foods, or do you consider them basically irrelevant to your therapy?

FL: Well, there are no direct links between foods and the immune system. However, essential amino acids play a primary role as precursors of noradrenaline and seratonin, the two neurotransmitters responsible for the immunoactivation and immuno suppression, respectively.

However, it is 'best' that people showing a high noradrenaline to adrenaline ratio should eat carbohydrates. Whereas, people showing a low noradrenaline to adrenaline ratio should eat mainly proteins.

Burzynski's Antineoplaston Therapy

Dr Stanislaw Burzynski has discovered cancer patients are missing certain chemical substances known as peptides. Naming them Antineoplastons, Burzynski has found that some of these peptides are particularly important in that they seem to form part of a biochemical defence the body mounts against cancerous cells (as opposed to an immune defence). Further, Dr Burzynski has gained immense experience in using Antineoplastons clinically, as for many years he has run a cancer clinic in Houston, Texas, along with a sophisticated Antineoplaston chemical production plant. Moreover, he has published extensively in peer-reviewed journals and his results and treatments have been investigated and confirmed by many respected doctors and professionals.

In particular, Antineoplastons have been documented as extremely effective against certain brain cancers, as well as Lymphomas—though at his clinic Burzynski treats a whole range of different cancers. A recent study of children with low-grade astrocytomas produced the following outstanding results. (It should be noted that children with astrocytoma's would seem to be the most certain responders to Antineoplastons and that other cancers with other age groups may not show such positive results). The results were:

Complete response:	37.5%
Partial response:	25.0%
Stable disease:	37.5%
Progressive disease:	0%
Complete response + Partial response:	62.5%
Complete response + Partial response + Stable disease:	100%

With such positive results as these, you may be asking why Antineoplastons are not a mainstream cancer therapy? To answer this question fully you are recommended to read either The Burzynski Breakthrough by Thomas Elias or the relevant chapter in The Cancer Industry by Ralph Moss. However we can note that Dr Burzynski's struggle with the mainstream to prove his therapy has been long and arduous—yet despite the trials and tribulations, Dr Burzynski has won through and proved to many influential medical professionals that his Antineoplastons do indeed exert a significant anticancer effect. He predicts it is only a matter of time before Antineoplastons are given the true place they deserve, and are accepted as a therapy of first choice by conventional oncologists. For instance in 1997, Dr Burdick, a highly respected oncologist of twenty-seven years practice, conducted a review of a number of Burzynski's patient's case histories. Burdick writes:

> 'Such remission rates are far in excess of anything that I or anyone else has seen since research work on brain tumours began. It is very clear that the responses here are due to antineoplaston therapy and are not due to surgery, radiation or standard chemotherapy. It is also clear that oftentimes responses are slow to develop in these tumours, despite almost daily therapy with antineoplastons and that when antineoplaston therapy is stopped tumours may re-grow within a few months. The duration of these responses is long and meaningful.'[38]

Therapy available at:

Burzynski Clinic
9432 Old Katy Road, Suite 200
Houston, TX 77055

☎:   713-335-5697
🖷:   713-335-5699
Email: info@burzynskiclinic.com
Web: www.cancermed.com

Approximate cost of therapy:

If enrolled in a clinical trial: No charge (but only certain patients who fit FDA criteria can be accepted).

Treatment outside of clinical trial (various options):

- Approximate charge for oral antineoplastons + Buphenyl is US$6,000 (£3750) per month.

- Approximate charge for oral antineoplastons is US$2,000-US$4,000 (£1250-£2500) per month.

- Cost of providing intravenous antineoplaston treatment is around US$14,000 (£8750) per month.

Usual length of stay at clinic: two to three weeks. After this you will need to take medication home with you (charged at the same rates as listed above).

The above prices do not include accommodation or food—though the Burzynski clinic will gladly assist you to locate somewhere appropriate.

How to obtain the therapy: Contact the clinic to find out details and to find out if the therapy is appropriate for you.

Interview With Dr Burzynski (Antineoplastons)

Simon Kelly: Dr Burzynski, can you start by speaking a little about peptides. What are they and how do they play a role in what you have termed a 'biochemical defence against cancer'.

Dr Stanislaw Burzynski: Peptides are chains of amino acids. You probably know that amino acids are also the building blocks of proteins. The difference between peptides and proteins is simply the length of the chain of amino acids.

Insulin was the first protein to be synthesised. Insulin contains fifty-one amino acids and it was assumed that whatever is below fifty amino acids in content are peptides. Anything above fifty amino acids is called a protein.

SK: So a peptide is a chain of less than fifty amino acids—a simpler form of protein?

SB: That's correct, yes. We can also evaluate it by checking molecular weight. So it's assumed that the molecular weight of a peptide is below five thousand. Above five thousand—then it's a protein.

SK: Molecular weight—is that the equivalent of weighing the peptide or protein on a set of scales?

SB: That's right—molecular weight means how many times the molecule is heavier than hydrogen. If you have a molecular weight of five thousand (approximately five thousand in the case of insulin), it means that this molecule is five thousand times heavier than an atom of hydrogen. It's another way of classifying it.

SK: What role do peptides play—and what happens when a person starts to get low on peptides?

SB: Peptides play a variety of roles,for instance, many hormones are peptides and many antibiotics are peptides. Generally speaking, they transfer and encode information. We can compare them to words and sentences in our language.

In most languages there are between twenty to thirty letters. With amino acids (the building blocks of peptides), there are twenty of them. Amino acids can be compared in this way to letters. You will note that with the twenty-six letters of the alphabet, you can encode a lot of information in words and sentences.

We could say that peptides are more like words, and proteins more like sentences, or even paragraphs. However, through the encoding of information in them, information about cancer is able to move from one part of the body to another.

SK: That's a very illuminating analogy.

SB: The peptides I discovered, and named antineoplastons, work as molecular switches. They carry information that is necessary to turn on certain genes that protect us against cancer—these genes are called tumour suppressor genes.

They also carry information that turn off genes that are causing cancer—these are called oncogenes. This means that we are able to turn off cancer growth accelerators and instead activate the brakes. But, if you don't have enough of these substances, then your body will be unable to turn on good genes and turn off bad genes—and then you may develop cancer.

SK: Basically, what you're saying is that you're working in a communications area.

SB: Information transfer inside the body—and this information is like a switch. Just as with other switches, you can turn on the engine of a car or even the engine of a jet—when we turn on the right switch, then we are increasing the activity of tumour suppressor genes. When we turn off the oncogene switch then it's like turning off electricity inside malignant cell. The cell will stop growing and die.

SK: Cells receive these pieces of information, carry the 'words' deep inside themselves, and then act upon them?

SB: That's right, yes. The mechanism of action has been identified so we know the chemical reactions that take place inside cells when antineoplastons are doing their job.

SK: You can follow the process of the peptide 'words' being processed inside the cell. But what is cancer and how does it begin?

SB: Cancer is a disease that arises because of the manufacturing of cells. Every day we have to manufacture millions of cells because we are continuously replacing cells in our body. For instance, in a single year, we are replacing eighteen livers and maybe exchanging eight urinary bladders etc. Within the time period of seven years, physically, every person becomes a new individual, because we have a complete set of new cells (except for brain cells and certain muscle cells that are not exchanged).

This means that there are tremendous manufacturing problems. As we have said, everyday we have to manufacture millions of new cells, and each of these cells consist of millions of different proteins, and each of the proteins consist of hundreds of amino acids that are in turn built out of numerous atoms of carbon, oxygen, nitrogen and hydrogen.

There's a tremendous problem of quality control and, statistically, one cell out of ten thousand will develop in the wrong way. Therefore the body must have a mechanism that will get rid of such cells. That is the system of antineoplastons. Antineoplastons activate tumour suppressor genes and tumour suppressor genes will force these abnormal cells to die.

Everyone develops cancer cells in their body—every day. But most of us are not getting cancer because we have a protective system consisting of antineoplastons and tumour suppressor genes, which force these abnormal cells to die.

However, when the system fails—when for instance, we don't have enough antineoplastons in our body or when we have a blockage or a mutation of tumour suppressor genes—then we develop cancer.

SK: That's a good explanation but why do we have tumour-promoting genes?

SB: Tumour-promoting genes are a normal part of our body and are necessary for the cells to grow.

In the cell system, they're under very strict control. They are only turned on for a very short time and then they are turned off again.

However, within cancer cells they are turned on all the time. That's why the assembly line, which is making these cells, is running all the time—making these defective cells.

SK: When a person becomes short of antineoplastons, what's happened—is it a dietary problem—is it an organ problem? Why the shortage?

SB: There are various problems that can contribute to it. For instance, maybe there's a mutation of the genes caused by external factors such as radiation or toxic chemicals—even stress. The genes that are responsible for synthesis of antineoplastons may have mutated—meaning that they don't make antineoplastons anymore.

SK: Where in the body are antineoplastons made—is there an area of the body where they are produced?

SB: We see them in a number of tissues in the body, in various quantities. We detect the highest concentration in the liver and in the kidneys. But this does not mean that they are made just in the liver and the kidneys, they are probably made in a variety of tissues in the body.

Further there are two types of antineoplastons, ones that have a broad spectrum of activity and work on a great variety of tissues—and other types that have a specific activity for specific tissue.

It is most likely that specific activity antineoplastons are produced in the cells of particular tissues—and that broad-spectrum antineoplastons are produced in the liver or kidneys.

If a person doesn't have enough antineoplastons in their body, then cancer cells can begin multiplying—and when there are a good number of cancer cells, they in turn will force the kidneys to eliminate even more antineoplastons from the body.

That's what happens with cancer patients. We see it, they eliminate a lot of antineoplastons in their urine, but they have none or very little in their blood. It's like a vicious circle in that the person with cancer is not able to make enough antineoplastons, and at the same time they are eliminating those they have produced.

SK: Why do you think that they are being eliminated—what's making that happen?

SB: Because cancer cells produce certain protein factors that instruct the kidneys to eliminate antineoplastons.

SK: Cancer cells always seem so sophisticated in their ability to paralyse the body's immune system (see p.34 for discussion of this point). But what about the huge increase in the incidence of cancer in recent decades—what do you think is causing this?

SB: We are living less and less healthy lives. We are surrounded by thousands of chemicals which can produce mutations or blockage of the genes. Dietary factors are also very important, for instance too much sugar and the resulting diabetes may produce blockage of the genes that are responsible for protecting us against cancer. Cigarette smoke, of course, is known to block the genes that protect against cancer.

On the other hand, we are diagnosing more cancer than ever before—for instance, because of the use of mammograms, we are detecting too many cancers. Some of these are medical mistakes and some of these are cancers at such an early stage that they may disappear without the intervention of medicine. This is the phenomenon we are seeing at the present time—we are over diagnosing breast cancer, we are over diagnosing prostate cancer.

SK: Let's take a look at how you initially discovered these peptides you have named antineoplastons. I read that you were using a technique called chromatography.

SB: At that time in the lab I used paper chromatography and thin layer chromatography. I was studying amino acids in the blood of healthy individuals and people with various illnesses, among them people who had cancer.

I discovered some substances that had not yet been identified. Some researchers from the University of Leeds, in the UK, had also already observed these substances but nobody had really attempted to identify them.

I thought it would be a good idea to identify them, because I was approaching the defence of my doctoral thesis, and I was afraid that I would be asked questions about these unknown substances.

I found the substances were indeed peptides and also that they were deficient in patients with cancer.

There was an obvious connection between the quantity of peptides in blood, and cancer. That's why I decided to isolate these peptides initially from blood (and later from urine), and test them in various tissue cultures of cancer cells and normal cells.

I found that at least some of them produced substantial inhibition of the growth of cancers, without effecting normal cells. It was remarkable at the time because the only chemicals that were known to inhibit cancer growth were very toxic chemotherapy drugs.

SK: How did you feel when you observed this?

SB: Obviously this was a great feeling though I was not the first person to find anti-cancer activity. At that time I was Professor at the Baylor College of Medicine, in Houston and I gave samples of the peptides to the researchers at the M.D. Andersen Cancer Centre. They tested them in various cancer models and also found strong anti cancer activity.

SK: Since then you have had twenty-five years experience using these peptides against cancer—what do you feel you can say about them, in terms of what they are good for and what they're not so useful for?

SB: Of course, we're not just talking about a single medicine. We have now developed twelve different formulations of antineoplastons and each has a different spectrum of activity. We have concentrated our efforts on using synthetic antineoplastons—not because they have the highest activity, but because this is the simplest way to produce them and also the simplest way to obtain FDA approval for clinical trials.

We have known from the beginning that the antineoplastons we are using don't work on every cancer. Therefore we have concentrated on the types of cancer which are the most difficult to treat. At the present time we have evidence coming from clinical trials supervised by the FDA, which proves anti-cancer activity in various types of brain tumours.

Some of the best results are those in the treatment of childhood brain tumours such as astrocytoma. It's a very common tumour in children and is practically incurable except for some sporadic cases where surgery is successful. We have also had good success with brainstem tumours. Normally, they are practically incurable because of their location in the brainstem.

Another indication for our treatment is a type of tumour called high grade gliomas which are malignant brain tumours that occur in adult patients— we have had very good results.

All of this is confirmed by studies of large numbers of patients under very scrutinised conditions. We have constant supervision by the FDA and experts from the FDA have reviewed the results of our treatment. So we are sure that we are right in this area.

Clinical trials in Japan have concentrated on the treatment of colon cancer with liver involvement as well as primary liver cancer. Antineoplastons have proved effective in these two types of cancer. The Japanese proved that antineoplastons have substantial activity in lung cancer, breast cancer and pancreatic cancer.

We see very good results in malignant lymphoma and prostate cancer. There are encouraging results in kidney cancer and cancer of the oesophagus and the stomach. At this time, we are treating seventy different types of cancer. However, in some of these groups we only have a small number of patients so we don't have statistics yet.

Antineoplastons work on the genes and it maybe that the same genes are involved in breast cancer, prostate cancer, brain tumour, pancreatic cancer, colon cancer, but in different percentages.

For instance in brain tumours, certain genes are involved in about seventy-five percent of patients. In breast cancer they may be involved in about twenty percent of patients who are of Caucasian origin—but in oriental patients, about fifty to sixty percent involvement. It is very helpful to know in advance which genes are involved in a particular patient.

We are now able to do such an analysis, for example, in a limited sense we can now detect, based on blood tests, the presence of some oncogenes that are more active. We are introducing methods that will give us very good information about nearly all the tumour suppressor genes and oncogenes that are involved in an individual patient's cancer. We are in the process of introducing this technology in our laboratory. We are confident that within a few months it will be in place.

SK: You are going to be able to work at the genetic level more precisely?

SB: That's correct. During the course of treatment we can repeat the test and find out if, for instance, the tumour suppressor genes that were blocked before the treatment started are now active (e.g. after the first month of treatment).

This is what medicine will be about in the next ten years. When a patient comes to the doctor, the doctor will be concerned not so much with how the cancer looks under the microscope, but what genes are involved.

SK: That's an interesting perspective.

SB: We are switching form the old classical knowledge of cancer that is based on its appearance under the optical microscope. This is quite outdated now and what we are more interested in is not what the cancer looks like under a microscope, but what kind of genes are involved? The genes will help us decide if the treatment will work or not.

SK: Let's go through what happens when a patient comes to you—do you consult with people over the phone first?

SB: Yes, one of our departments talks with the patient extensively. If necessary, the patient can talk to one of our doctors—we have about twenty-five doctors who work in the clinic. Then, if we feel that we can help the patient, we ask them to come for a consultation.

Many patients contact us from places a long way away & because they have some of the toughest cases of cancer, we don't want them to travel all the way to Houston to then find we aren't able to accept them. That's why we like to predetermine if there's a chance that treatment may work.

SK: Are people able to come for treatment from abroad?

SB: Yes, quite a few patients come from abroad. We prefer to make contact with the doctor who will take care of the patient in their home country, and when the patient returns home, we send a letter to their doctor, outlining further treatment.

SK: Is it correct that the first procedure a patient has to undergo is the placing of a catheter into their chest?

SB: Not necessarily, it depends whether the patient qualifies for admission to clinical trials—and only some patients qualify. The majority do not—the rules were introduced by the FDA.

In the average month, we have approximately eight hundred people who would like to come for treatment. Out of these, perhaps only ten or twenty qualify for clinical trials. The rest of the patients are treated outside clinical trials.

By chance, it happens that a medicine approved by the FDA for a different purpose (for the treatment of liver failure) is metabolised into one of our antineoplastons inside a patient's liver.

This means that patients who qualify for this type of treatment don't need to be treated within a clinical trial. We can simply prescribe for them, this medicine that is already approved by the FDA. This treatment is given orally in tablets.

The majority of patients, (I would say about eighty percent of patients), are taking these tablets or capsules outside of clinical trials. Some of these patients also use chemotherapy or immunotherapy—whatever is the best for the individual patient. It's only a minority of patients who are treated in clinical trials—and most of these patients will receive intravenous antineoplastons. This means they need a placement of an intravenous catheter so that the medicines can be delivered using a pump.

SK: I'm wondering if patients might feel they are receiving a second best treatment if they don't qualify for treatment within a clinical trial.

SB: Well, it has advantages and disadvantages. With treatment taking place within clinical trials, we are giving large doses of antineoplastons. The FDA usually reserve this type of treatment for patients who have very advanced with stage four disease and/or patients who have already failed various other treatments. Not everybody requires such intensive treatment. Also, for those being treated within clinical trials, we are not able to add any additional treatments such as immunotherapy.

SK: Going back to the name of the FDA approved medicine you mentioned— what is the name of that medicine?

SB: It's called Buphenyl. It was introduced for the treatment of liver failure in children, but there's only a very small population of such patients. Within the entire United States, there is thought to be less than three hundred. Therefore the medicine is not well known, but since we are carrying out research in this area, we became aware that a team from John Hopkin's

Medical School had identified that this medicine is converted into one of our antineoplastons inside the liver.

SK: Probably you would prefer to be treating all your patients in the same way as those being treated within clinical trials.

SB: I would prefer to treat patients out of the clinical trial framework because it is very difficult.

Within clinical trials, we have to submit weekly reports to the FDA and we have to submit monthly reports and we have to submit annual reports. The bureaucracy is tremendous. We have to employ something like twenty people just to take care of bureaucracy for these clinical trials.

SK: You have to spend a lot of time form filling?

SB: Oh, it's horrible. After we have seen patients for a couple of months there are already two thousand pages. If we don't do it right, then they can suspend clinical trials. Last year they suspended two hundred clinical trials at John Hopkin's Medical School, because of some discrepancies.

The government also determines how many blood tests patients should have per week, how soon a scan needs to be done. This is tedious for us and tedious for the patients.

The government requires that in the first two months of treatment, a patient should have three blood tests a week—at least, whether they need it or not. And because they have decided in Washington that patients should have so many blood tests per week, there is nothing we can do. We have to obey the orders and do it—but if I would treat patients in my private practice...

SK: ... You wouldn't do it quite the same way. You mentioned combining antineoplastons with other treatments. Can you say a bit more about that?

SB: It depends—with brain tumours, antineoplastons work best when you leave them alone, without any additional treatments. The same with prostate cancer and malignant lymphoma.

However, with advanced breast cancer that has spread throughout the patients entire body, much better results are obtained if we combine antineoplaston-producing medication like Buphenyl with hormonal treatment, or with immunotherapy.

In lung cancer patients, we get better results if we combine antineoplastons with some form of chemotherapy—but given in a way so the patient does not expereince adverse reactions.

That's what we are using now, but in the future we will be introducing additional antineoplastons, which will probably eliminate the need for additional treatments such as chemotherapy.

We have developed many antineoplastons but we are not allowed to use them because of FDA restrictions. The rules require us to go through a whole series of clinical trials for each new antineoplaston—but this is something which is very difficult for us to afford. The patients who are in clinical trials receive the treatment for free—we don't charge them for the medicine. This means, every patient enrolled in a clinical trial, costs us thousands of dollars (from our own pockets).

SK: How many useful types of antineoplastons are there?

SB: We have developed (and already tested on animals and humans) twelve pharmaceutical formulations. But in addition to these, there are at least another thirty we have discovered. We are in the process of developing the second and third generation of antineoplastons, which have about a thousand times more activity compared to the ones we are using now.

SK: You feel that these offer great promise—if only you could start using them?

SB: You're right, yes—but it is a tedious process. In the United States it costs a lot of money to develop a medicine. To develop one single medicine, the cost is in the area of five hundred million dollars. Really, it's very difficult to afford it. We are generating a significant amount of money in our private practice, but it goes almost entirely into developing new antineoplastons. Without this private income we wouldn't be able to exist, because we don't receive any grants from the government and are developing entirely from our own financial resources.

SK: As we are speaking about money, can we discuss the costs for a patient treated outside clinical trials.

SB: The majority of patients will pay around $6,000 (£3750) per month, because they will take Buphenyl. Because this is an FDA approved medicine, health insurances are paying for a good percentage of these patients.

If a patient has intravenous infusions of antineoplastons, the equipment to do it such as the pump, various supplies, nursing services and doctor's services, usually comes to around approximately $14,000 (£8750) per month. Again, insurance companies usually meet the costs.

Regarding treatment with antineoplaston capsules—this comes to between $2,000 and $4,000 (£1250-£2500) per month.

Patients enrolled in clinical trails need to stay between two to three weeks. Patients being treated outside clinical trials typically stay for one to two weeks. Then treatment continues under the care of their local physician.

On top of this patients need to budget for hotel and living costs.

SK: How long do patients need to continue treatment?

SB: We advise the patient to continue treatment for at least eight months after there are no more signs of cancer—just to eliminate any microscopic cancer cells in the body (which may not be detectable via scans).

SK: Changing subject slightly, can you say a little about the new supplement you have just released.

SB: We have obtained FDA approval for a supplement, and have begun to market it this year. It's available in the United States and Europe.

SK: How does this supplement fit in, for instance, it contains antineoplastons, but you are not marketing it for cancer. You are marketing it as a health supplement—possibly a preventative.

SB: It's a supplement that contains of a number of amino acids, and these amino acids do have anti cancer activity. It also contains vitamin B2, which has anti cancer activity at certain dosages—and it contains A10, one of our own antineoplaston preparations, in small dosages.

Scientific experiments carried out in Japan and the Medical College of Georgia in the United States, demonstrate we can prevent occurrences of lung, breast and liver cancer when we add a small amount of the supplement preparation to animal food (and expose the animals to carcinogens).

Based on this finding, our advice is for people to take one capsule twice a day or two capsules twice a day, depending on body weight. It has also been shown to decrease the toxic effects of chemotherapy—so patients who are receiving chemotherapy will notice the benefits of taking it.

More and more people are using the product, and, we are also introducing some additional products like cosmetic cream—which will protect people from the development of skin cancer.

SK: What value does the supplement have for people already have cancer? Obviously it's not as strong as your specific cancer treatment preparations.

SB: It's not strong enough to control advanced cancer, but it's helpful as a complementary treatment (to say chemotherapy). It may reduce the toxicity of chemotherapy and increase its effectiveness. We have some reports form a Dutch oncologist who has given patients the supplement plus chemotherapy. They have reported very good results.

SK: How you see the future of cancer therapy developing—do you see a cure in the near future?

SB: Oh, certainly—we already have the answer to some types of cancer. I believe that within another twenty years the population will be screened to predetermine if you have, for instance, blockages or mutations of important genes that protect against cancer.

Individuals who have such blockages or mutations will receive the preventative formulations similar to what we are developing now. This will enable them to avoid cancer in the first place. And if a person does developed cancer, then we will be able to treat it effectively with medicines designed to affect particular genes.

SK: What about antineoplastons—do you see them becoming mainstream in the near future?

SB: Sure, yes. I believe that we can receive final approval for marketing antineoplastons within the next two to three years in the United States, and shortly thereafter for the European Community and Australia. But this is just the first step because, as I have mentioned, we are introducing newer formulations of antineoplastons that are more active, and in the future it won't be necessary to give injections of them—it will be much simpler.

SK: Dr Burzynski, you have already fought and won many important battles (with authorities such as the FDA) and yet it sounds like you're just beginning.

SB: Certainly, yes. If you compare it to the development of planes, we are probably at the level of a DC3 aeroplane—there are a lot of improvements that can be made.

It is not only our team that is working intensively in this area, but also many other teams in the world. Of course, most of them are working completely independently from us—because the time is now approaching that this will be proved the right treatment for cancer.

SK: I am wondering about the last twenty-five years of your life—with the discovery of antineoplastons, beginning to produce them, the court cases and everything that has been thrown at you by the authorities—how did you keep your head?

SB: Well now, you see, I knew that I was right—and it helps, because when you are right then why should you submit to people who really don't understand what you are doing?

I have simply provided evidence that I am using the right approach. It's like, for instance, if you went back in time and used penicillin for the treatment of pneumonia. Other people might kill you for it, because they would say that you are doing witchcraft.

SK: But how did you keep your head with all those court cases? They went on for years, with charges that would have sent you to prison for three hundred years. That must have been an enormous pressure—or did you somehow just let it wash over you?

SB: At the time I was working long hours. For instance I usually woke up at around four in the morning—and would come to the office very early because I needed to see patients before I went to court at eight in the morning.

Then I would come back to my office at around 5 pm and see more patients. Then I went to sleep at around eleven or twelve. There was no time for anything else—I had to survive.

SK: Your struggle is an inspiring and great story. It's as if you took one step at a time—but it's amazing how far you have travelled.

SB: That's correct. With such a powerful medical establishment and government support of the large pharmaceutical companies—there's no other way. You have to persist sometimes.

SK: Dr Burzynski, thank you for explaining about antineoplastons in such a clear and concise way.

SB: You're welcome. It's my pleasure.

Burton's Immuno-Augmentive Therapy

Lawrence Burton, a cancer researcher at New York University first made headlines in 1966, when, using his Immuno-Augmentative Therapy, he performed a demonstration in front of seventy scientists, two hundred writers and numerous press reporters. For the demonstration he used mice bearing large 'rock-hard' tumours. In front of the assembled audience, Burton injected the mice with his immune factor compounds and showed that, after an hour and a half, each of the mouse's immune systems had been stimulated to ferociously attack the tumours. Over the next few hours, the tumours literally melted away and disappeared in front of the assembled audience's eyes. Though of course this demonstration was with mice and not with humans, it was still an utterly astounding spectacle.

Many top scientists and researchers immediately cried foul, branded Burton a 'quack', and demanded the demonstrations be repeated. Burton obligingly repeated the demonstrations a while later in front of an audience of oncologists at the New York Academy of Medicine. As an added precaution, two other doctors performed the actual demonstration (rather than Burton), and members of the audience were able to choose which of sixteen mice they wanted to treat. Again the demonstration was successful, and again many cried foul. However, here are some reports from individuals who saw Burton's demonstrations close up.

Science writer for the Philadelphia Bulletin, David Cleary, reports:

> 'The two gentlemen from St. Vincent's Hospital demonstrated before our very eyes that injection of a mysterious serum ... caused the disappearance of massive tumours in mice within a few hours.'[39]

At a slightly later time, Patrick McGrady Sr, a well-respected American Cancer Society official, asked Burton for an impromptu demonstration of his methods while he was staying as a patient in the hospital where Burton carried out his research. He reports:

> 'I saw him perform miracles on those mice... He'd make the tumours disappear while you watched. There's no question in my mind that this was authentic.'[40]

Though Burton made it clear that what he had discovered wasn't a 'cure' for cancer, but rather an immune system augmenting (immune boosting) factor, it was still an important breakthrough. Burton worked hard to have his findings confirmed by other mainstream researchers, but unfortunately, the major cancer institutions (and their researchers) could not bring themselves to deal with Burton, a person they considered rude, vulgar and not suited to be a member of the establishment. Burton found himself isolated from mainstream research and so in 1977 he decided to take his laboratory to the Bahamas—where it remains to this day.

With reference to his demonstrations with the mice, Burton explained that his compounds 'de-blocked' their immune systems, thereby freeing them up and allowing them to attack the tumours. For some reason, at the time of the development of a tumour, a blocking protein is produced that 'blocks' optimal immune system functioning. Specifically, this blocking compound interferes with the feedback mechanism that is responsible for the release of tumour destroying compounds such as tumour necrosis factor.

Burton identified the working of this feedback mechanism, and isolated four specific compounds that work together to provide balance and control. By altering and manipulating the levels of these compounds Burton discovered he could reverse the immune system paralysis (caused by the tumour), and enable the natural tumour killing necrosis factors to resume their work. Though originally working with mice, Burton found the same immune system de-blocking techniques could be transferred across species to human beings.

In terms of practical application, Burton's therapy consists of first measuring the levels of various immune system hormones to ascertain how they exist in relation to each other. The levels are analysed via a formula that Burton formulated from many years of experience. Then, as indicated by the results of the analysis, the levels of the compounds are altered using injections of relevant factors.

The aim of the therapy is to lull tumour cells into a false sense of 'security' that they have paralysed the immune system—(when in fact they haven't done so at all), while at the same time restoring full working capability to the immune system.

At the IAT centre in Freeport, individuals receiving the therapy gather daily at 7.30 AM for a blood analysis. By 9.30, the analysis is complete and everyone receive and self-inject the correct level of IAT serum (indicated by Burton's formula). Individuals typically stay for an initial seven weeks, during which time the clinic can ascertain how well the therapy is working, as well as identify the make up of serum each individual will take home with them.

The clinic is located in a beautiful environment and is renowned for its uplifting psychosocial atmosphere. You can find out more about the therapy and the clinic in the interview contained below with John Clement—IAT's director.

Therapy available at:

IAT (Bahamas) Ltd.
P.O. Box F-42689
Freeport
Grand Bahama
Bahamas
☎:   (242) 352-7455
🖷:   (242) 352-3201
E-mail: burtonh101@aol.com
Web: www.iatclinic.com

Cost of therapy:

First month: £4687 (US$7500).

Per week after first month: £437.50 (US$700).

Average stay at clinic: six to ten weeks/average eight weeks.

Cost of take home medications: £31.25 (US$50) per week.

Accommodation and food is not included—though the clinic will help you find somewhere reasonably priced.

How to go about receiving the therapy: Contact the IAT clinic to find out if the therapy is suitable for your particular cancer.

Interview With John Clement (Burton's IAT Therapy)

Former colleague of Dr Burton, Dr John Clement became manager of the IAT clinic after Dr Burton's death in 1993. Dr Clement worked with Dr Burton for many years and was intimately acquainted with Burton's work and ideas, as well as being a close personal friend.

Simon Kelly: Hello John—thank you for agreeing to discuss the IAT clinic you have run since Lawrence Burton died in 1993. Can we begin with a brief outline of the treatments you are offering?

Dr John Clement: At the present time we're offering two therapies. Our main therapy is Burton's Immune Augmentation Therapy (which we have optimised considerably over the years). The basic theory still stands, but we've got better at making the serum and we've got better at administering it. We are also offering a tumour specific dendritic cell vaccine.

SK: Can you describe Burton's therapy in more detail? Most summaries of the treatment explain that Burton's therapy works via an immune system de-blocking protein. Can we go through the theory of the treatment in a little more detail?

JC: Way back, researchers started investigating cytokines. (Definition of cytokines: regulatory proteins released by cells of the immune system that act as intercellular mediators in the generation of an immune response.)

One of the cytokines Burton started working on is now called Tumour Necrosis Factor. He found that with this factor, he could kill cancer cells. He found he could do it in-vitro, and in-vivo, and that he could even cross species with it. This means that, in their body, every person has a system of scavenging cancer cells, but it appears that something can go wrong with the mechanism, and, if it does go wrong, then a person is no longer able to control outbreaks of cancer cells.

SK: So what specifically goes wrong with tumour necrosis factor in the cancer patient? Is it the levels of it?

JC: Well, when you use these tumour necrosis factors to kill cells (there are several different tumour necrosis factors), cell death is recognised by the body as something wrong. The body knows that if there are too many cells being killed, there's the danger that the body will experience toxicity problems. Because of this, the body produces a protein, a blocking protein. Now, this is the theory of Burton's—he said, 'If there is a blocking protein being produced, then we must try and remove it'.

SK: You're describing that the body needs to regulate the tumour necrosis factors for various reasons, and to do this, it uses certain blocking proteins. At the same time, however, that the body regulates the working of tumour necrosis factors—it runs the risk of not eliminating cancers.

JC: That's right—and Burton looked for a way of stopping the blocking protein.

SK: Burton aimed to block the blocking protein itself, thereby freeing up the tumour necrosis factors to kill the cancer.

JC: Burton reasoned that if he used a substance of similar molecular weight to tumour necrosis factor, that it might act as a decoy. And Burton did indeed find that when he used this similar molecular weighted molecule that he could stop the blocking protein. We call it a de-blocking protein. It blocks the blocking protein.

SK: So Burton's therapy works by exerting an effect further up in the bodies control hierarchy—and that the effect of this is that it leads to more tumour necrosis factor being released or available.

I am recalling that conventional medicine also discovered Tumour Necrosis Factor (TNF) at a later date, (of interest is that unconventional cancer therapy critic Saul Green was a member of the team that discovered TNF on the conventional side—and that he became Burton's chief enemy and critic). What is the link between the two applications of TNF?

JC: What happened is that conventional medicine tried [to use TNF for therapeutic purposes] but they didn't come up with idea of the blocking protein. Without taking into account the blocking protein, what happens is, that the more necrosis factor you give, the more toxic it becomes to the patient.

You kill a little bit of tumour with the first dose, a little bit more with the next larger dose—and with a vastly increased dose, maybe a fraction more of the tumour—but then if you go the whole hog, there is a likelihood the patient will die.

Tumour necrosis factor is highly toxic and conventional medicine didn't discover or didn't think of the fact that maybe another factor or two are involved (i.e. the de-blocking protein).

Whereas, in contrast, Burton reasoned, 'There's got to be a factor produced which is causing the tumour necrosis factor to stop working'.

SK: So conventional doctors give more and more tumour necrosis factor to the patient, but unfortunately it has more and more diminishing returns in terms of killing the tumour, while at the same time being very toxic to the patient?

But how does Burton's IAT therapy get around the toxicity of the tumour necrosis factor? Surely to kill the cancer, the level of tumour necrosis factor has to increase as well?

JC: Well no, we're not increasing the level of TNF drastically, we don't have to. What they failed to recognise was the fact that they were giving larger doses to the patients and that the blocking protein was just stopping it working.

SK: This seems a very important point, can you reiterate it.

JC: Without our therapy, the blocking factor neutralises the tumour necrosis factor and so the dose has to be continually increased, (for some TNF to be available to fight the cancer). This non-availability is due to the fact that it is being blocked.

SK: So, at the risk of labouring the point, what you're saying is that conventional doctors give lots of tumour necrosis factor, but it never really works on the cancer because of it being continually blocked by the blocking protein. But in addition, even though the tumour necrosis factor is being blocked in terms of its action against the tumour cells, the patients expereinces toxicity due to the large amounts of TNF present in their body.

So is the blocking protein working on a local basis around the tumour?

JC: We don't know where it comes from or what produces it, but it's there, and unless it's neutralised—then larger and larger doses of tumour necrosis factor don't do any good. We prevent that blocking from happening.

Some years after Burton had discovered all this a researcher called Rick Lentz speculated, 'If Burton is right, and there is a blocking protein, we should be able to remove the blocking protein completely from the patient, and then patients will be able to kill their own cancer'.

This was very interesting work because his hypothesis was that the blocking protein must be similar to a protein factor found in pregnant mammals. Pregnant mammals, of course, have in them, a body which is not them (i.e. a foetus).

The body in them (the foetus) can be a different colour, race, creed, blood group, everything. But pregnant mammals don't usually abort their own foetus. There are a lot of similarities to cancer in this.

SK: You're suggesting that a pregnant mammal is utilising the same blocking process to stop it attacking the growing foetus as may be happening in the person with cancer?

JC: That's right—and Lentz discovered (and isolated) the blocking protein in pregnant goats. He said, 'if we could remove that, then we would have it made', because, 'maybe then we could remove the blocking protein from humans'.

Eventually they made a kidney membrane, which could remove the blocking protein from animals or people. They carried out research on goats and found that if they removed the blocking protein, that the animal did indeed abort. Further, if they gave it back before the animal aborted, it would stop the abortion process.

They then tried taking the blocking protein from one goat and giving it to another goat, and they found that it crossed between animals—and then they found that it crossed species and eventually got to the state where they were prepared to dialyse a patient to remove the blocking protein. Lentz even got FDA approval to treat a number of people.

Through the people he treated Lentz proved that he had a viable way of killing tumours by self-rejection. It was at this stage that he came to Burton. The problem Lentz had was that he couldn't tell how fast he was removing the blocking protein—but Burton had already figured out how to measure this.

We thought we would dialyse patients here in Freeport but we never got round to it because Burton died and Lentz ran out of money. But I've heard that he's back doing it again now.

SK: I am wondering how what we have discussed here is applied to modern day IAT therapy in practice?

JC: Well, we take patient's blood daily—just a very small amount and measure the level of the various tumour necrosis factors in it. In addition, we measure the amount of blocking protein present.

Then we give back (to the patient) de-blocking protein and tumour necrosis factor at the precise level necessary for therapeutic effect. We negate the effect of the blocking protein and add in small amounts of the killing factor. We do this via a series of injections, each day.

It's not quite as simple as that because we also measure other factors that relate to the patient's own immune system, because we are attempting to augment that whole system. We can produce massive [tumour] kills, but at the expense of augmenting the patient's own immune system.

SK: You mean you have to be careful not to sideline a patient's own immune system?

JC: Yes—we can really override the patient's own immune system if we want to, but then the moment we stop treating we find that we've thrown their whole body out of balance and things are likely to get worse rapidly.

SK: It sounds as if the process needs to be very subtle to have a good long-term therapeutic effect.

JC: Yes it is a very subtle process and the amounts of treatment we are giving are minute—down to a molecular level.

SK: Changing subject slightly, what about when someone comes to you with cancer, what is your process—how do you decide whether you're going to be able to help them?

JC: First before they come they must have had a full pathological diagnosis and we need to see a full report about the kind of cancer they've got, and the treatments they've already received.

If the cancer is surgically removable, then it must be operated on before they come.

SK: You consider the removal of a tumour outweighs any risks of disturbing the cancer, possibly causing metastases? (Some commentators are concerned about the risk of spilling cancer cells into the rest of the body during surgery or biopsies).

JC: Yes—the lower the tumour burden you've got to work on, the better response you are going to get.

SK: Let us say a person has come to you, and that they've had their tumour removed and that they also have a good diagnosis in the sense that it is known exactly what the type of cancer is—what happens next?

JC: We would start treating them to see what response we get. If we get a response, it indicates that they probably still have a tumour (i.e. that some cancer is left in their body).

SK: On average, could you say how many people do respond positively to the treatment (in terms of a regression of their cancer). Is it, say, fifty percent—or more or less?

JC: No, most people do respond—it's very, very rare that we get no response.

Actually we hope that we prevent people who are likely to have no response from coming to the clinic in the first place. For instance, people who have had very extensive chemotherapy, or who are in extremely poor health. And the other kind of person we are unable to treat, I'm afraid, are people who have had bone marrow transplants.

SK: Because their immune systems have been subjected to such an onslaught?

JC: Yes.

SK: And people stay, I have heard, for an initial period of about ten weeks?

JC: Well, six to ten, yes. The average is probably about eight. We test patient's blood about eight times a week, and based on the results of these, we give them IAT serum shots (to give to themselves). Each shot is less than half a cc and they are given with the finest insulin syringes, you can barely feel the needle going in.

SK: Can you say a bit more about the results you have obtained with IAT?

JC: We've had a lot of excellent results. At the moment I know we've got two women here with mesothelioma on both lungs, and they are both doing incredibly well—mesothelioma, as you know, is a ghastly cancer caused by asbestos.

We've had more success with this cancer than anywhere else in the world. Some years ago, the National Foundation for Alternative Medicine set themselves the task of travelling to various clinics around the world that are offering alternative therapies, to document what each of them do.

They came to us early on—about eight people came here for about a week with two medical statisticians. They went through our records and found twenty cases in which there were abnormal results that could be attributed to our treatment rather than anything else.

They produced two volumes of case histories of these twenty best cases—mesothelioma figured prominently.

SK: Which other cancers are other good responders to IAT treatment?

JC: Doctors quite often send people who dealing with colon cancer that has metastasised to their liver. For instance we have a patient, who is in fact an MD in America—he came here four years ago with colon cancer, which had metastasised to his liver. His liver is now clear.

SK: What about breast cancer in women?

JC: Breast cancer—it's variable because they come in so many different stages. Generally, however, we have had luck with almost all the breast cancers except the inflammatory breast cancers. An inflammatory breast cancer is like it says, it's like an abscess—the breast rots away at a furious rate—it's a rapidly growing cancer.

SK: What would you say to people with cancer? What would your advice be to someone struggling with decisions about which treatment direction they should take?

JC: My guru for all these things is Ralph Moss. Many people, including doctors, would do well reading his book Questioning Chemotherapy.

It's an unbiased, descriptive account of chemotherapy. Ralph Moss is a most meticulous person—he doesn't put anything down on paper unless he has verified it.

SK: We agree—we are suggesting readers with cancer invest in one of Ralph Moss's individualised reports so they can familiarise themselves with the statistical chance offered to them by conventional treatments.

Going back one stage to Burton's therapy again. I would like you to explain in more detail about what has happened to the patient's body—why is the cancer patient producing immune system blocking proteins—what has gone out of balance?

JC: A lot of people have suggested that a situation occurs in the body where little nests of cells start behaving abnormally. Usually, these cells are sanitised by tumour necrosis factor; however, there comes a point when this nest of cells grows to about the size of a pinhead, that it becomes self-supporting. It may be this moment that the blocking factor starts being produced and which in turn prevents tumour necrosis factor from killing the cells. Once this happens, the tumour is out of control in terms of the body's natural defences.

SK: Once the nest of cancer cells achieves a critical mass and is able to start producing the blocking compound they just go off on their own.

JC: The mass is awfully small. When the surgeon says, 'I got everything' he means he's got everything he could see—and to be quite honest, what he can't see, are things the size of a pinhead.

SK: A very direct question now—do you really feel that you can help people with this therapy? Ralph Moss was explaining me his view, that it is difficult to evaluate how effective alternative cancer clinics are, because so often a 'cure', can actually be put down to a previously received conventional treatment. He feels that many people who attend clinics such as yours, are actually attending for reasons of secondary prevention—and that it is very difficult to ascertain whether they would have experienced a reoccurrence if they had decided not to visit an alternative cancer clinic.

JC: Yes, but in terms of the IAT clinic, almost all the people who receive treatment come because they have reoccurrences. Individuals who have had chemotherapy and seem to be well, aren't the kind of people who come to us. People come to us when they get problems.

SK: From your perspective then, you see the therapy really does help people?

JC: Oh, yes.

SK: And in terms of the treatment, do you aim to completely eliminate the tumour—or is it more common that the tumour stabilises?

JC: This is the same thing. We have a lady who is coming back next week—she had a renal cell carcinoma about twenty-two years ago.

The renal cell cancer was removed, but it had metastasised to her lungs and liver (at the time these metastasises were biopsied). This lady received IAT treatment, but on a CAT scan you can still see the metastasises in her lungs and her liver.

Her doctors contend that the previously reported metastasises are artefacts (meaning that they're something—but that they were not cancer). But we have the original biopsy results, so we know that they were cancer. This is what happens with our treatment, very often we can kill the tumour and it's left sitting there—dead.

SK: I have heard that the environment is very strong and supportive at the clinic—very conducive to healing

JC: Yes, for instance at the moment we have some returnees—some old patients coming back for check ups—it's a bit like a club. I think that helps the treatment, but I don't think that makes it, you can't cure lung cancer with a nice trip.

SK: You don't think that the social environment is responsible for the cure, but it helps?

JC: I think it's naïve to think that because a place is nice that it's going to cure cancer. But, I think the patients are terribly helpful to each other. When you come here, you meet a lot of people, you meet a woman of thirty-nine who was told she was dying when she was eight years old. Patients see this gorgeous creature walking around giving everybody a hug, saying, 'You know, just stick with it'.

We've got two women (women aren't supposed to have mesothelioma), and both are doing incredibly well—and of course they're sharing that with everybody. There's all these people walking around who are doing well, and some of the people who are here now and who have been here a while are very positive. All that helps. But you've got to have something that works to start it off.

SK: For a patient, speaking to someone who's had a positive result from the therapy and is still alive—is going to mean an incredible amount in terms of morale and motivation.

JC: Yes. We've got an old lady of eighty-four—she's been coming here for eight or nine years now. Her son comes down with her because she's not particularly good at travelling anymore. I saw the son and I said, 'You know, your mother doesn't really have to come back anymore'. 'I know' he said, 'but she likes it, this is one of her treats'.

And the staff are absolutely loyal. All the staff have been here for years and they're all cross-trained, they can all do everything. All the lab staff are cross-trained and the office staff are quite capable of doing each other's jobs, which makes life very easy.

We're also now offering ILT, an immune, tumour specific dendritic cells cancer vaccine. It was originally produced by Aiden Laboratories but now it's being made here.

In my opinion we're not really alternative—we were using cytokines before people even knew what a cytokine was. At first, when Burton started, mainstream medicine hadn't yet discovered interferon. When he came along, they just didn't know what he was talking about.

SK: I'm wondering if we can just cover approximate costs?

JC: The cost of our treatment for the first month of treatment is US$7,500 (£4687). Thereafter, while the patient is here, it's $700 (£437.50) a week.

At first, after the patient returns home, the maintenance therapy they take with them is $50 (£31.25) a week. Generally, after the initial stay, patients come back sixteen weeks later, usually for about ten days. During this return period, we test them on a daily basis to ensure what we're giving them is just right.

SK: If people are interested in coming to the IAT clinic for treatment, I understand you will give them an indication over the telephone as to whether you think it is worth them coming?

JC: Yes, that's right. If we're doubtful as to whether we can help, we will accept a patient for a two-week trial, (for which we will charge half the monthly amount).

SK: You mentioned you that can ascertain quite quickly the kind of response an individuals body is going to have in respect to the treatment.

JC: We can pretty well tell whether we're having any effect. But we can't tell whether it's a completely good effect at that stage.

SK: Let's say a patient's come and they're getting a response, a good response— what can you tell from that? For instance, can you say, 'I think we're going to be able to save your life'—or are there still too many unknowns?

JC: We wouldn't say that—we don't claim we cure or save life. We just say, 'Look, we're helping'. Even to people who have survived twenty years—we say, 'Well, you're lucky—but just remember you're a cancer patient'.

I think that anybody who's had cancer has got to do that.

SK: You're emphasising the need to take good care of themselves?

That feels like a good point to finish on. We have covered some important points as to how IAT therapy works—and you have given us a good feel of the clinic and what you can offer. Thank you very much John.

JC: And thank you too.

Cellular Light Therapy (CLT) & Photodynamic Therapy (PDT)

Introductory note: We are aware, that in the interest of our readers protection, some commentators might consider it more prudent for us to leave out this section on PDT/CLT. This is because over the last year, PDT/CLT has caused a lot of controversy—a study did not show the benefit that many people had presumed it would, and there were several reports of individuals feeling they were not well treated by CLT Clinics of Ireland.

We feel, however that it is important you are provided with information about PDT/CLT, so that you can make your own choice as to whether to utilise the therapy (though if you choose to go the CLT route rather than one of the other similar PDT routes, we recommend you be extremely careful in dealing with CLT Clinics, and follow the advice we will detail later). Furthermore, the last year has seen several long standing (and professionally run) clinics begin offering the treatment to individuals with cancer and, the cost of treatment has come down slightly.

The principles of photodynamic therapy have been established for many decades, and are simple and straightforward—light is used to activate a photo-sensitive compound (either given orally, intravenously or applied directly to the skin), which has an ability to accumulate in cancer cells but not in normal healthy cells. As the photodynamic agent is activated by the light (usually at a very specific wavelength of light) it becomes excited, electrons in the agent molecules shift into higher orbits and/or are released—the end result being that singlet oxygen is created inside cancer cells. Singlet oxygen is very reactive, and tends to have the effect of impairing cancer cells—so they are not able to operate at full strength or undergo cellular division. For instance, singlet oxygen released inside a cell might damage its mitochondria—its energy producing centre.

A new generation of photodynamic cancer therapy agents have recently been developed. The new agents are known by the names CLT agent or Radachlorin and are attracting a significant amount of interest—as well as controversy. The development of these new agents has led to PDT type therapies becoming available to the public, outside of mainstream institutions. Up until 2002, PDT was only available for very specific cancers (e.g. certain head and neck cancers), at a few specialist medical centres around the world. Now however, there are a variety of offerings from various clinics, and it is possible the therapy will prove a useful addition to your therapeutic program—though CLT/PDT should be considered an experimental treatment in the sense that protocols for the newer agents are only just being worked out. You might also consider approaching your oncologist, and/or checking out cancer information services in your country to find out if conventional PDT is offered for your type of cancer.

The main limitation up until this time with PDT treatment has been due to the limitations of first generation photodynamic agents. To be of most value, the agent need to be taken up preferentially by cancer cells, rather than by normally functioning cells. If the photodynamic agent does *not* accumulate preferentially in cancer cells, then healthy cells are at risk of damage when they are exposed to light, just as much as cancer cells. First generation agents such as Photofrin only have a selectivity for cancer cells (as opposed to normal cells) of around 3:1 (i.e. three molecules of the agent accumulate in cancer cells compared with one in healthy cells). Second generation agents however, have selectivity for cancer cells in the range of 60:1 to 200:1.

Another problem stemming from the low selectivity of early generation agents (and the resulting accumulation in healthy cells as well as cancerous cells) is that they tend to remain active in the body for long periods of time after treatment—making normal life very difficult for people receiving therapy. For instance, Photofrin, remains active in the body for up to thirty days, and recipients of therapy need to keep themselves covered up and out of the sun for this period as they might easily contract severe sunburn. In contrast, the newer photosensitive agents are typically ninety five percent eliminated from the body after twenty-four hours.

The new second-generation photodynamic compounds are synthesised from natural compounds such as spirulina (a common algae, available in health stores) or seaweed, and if used appropriately and carefully, toxicity issues can be kept to a minimum. Though it is a simplification in terms of the biochemistry that takes place when the agent is illuminated by light, we can compare the process to the natural process of photosynthesis, where plants harvest the energy of the sun.

When the photosensitive agent is activated by laser light (of a specific wavelength), it produces singlet oxygen molecules, a powerful free radical which destroys or damages cancer cells by oxidation. The best outcome in terms of internal cancer cell damage is that it is sufficient enough to cause cells natural apoptotic (programmed cell death) functionality to 'kick-in'. In contrast, if too much agent or light is used then the amount of singlet oxygen created may cause cellular necrosis (drastic cell death)—which in turn is likely to lead to undesirable inflammation around the tumour. We should note that neither the photosensitive agent, nor the light, is able to damage or kill cancer cells on their own—rather it is the combination of the two that is responsible for therapeutic action.

What is the difference between PDT and CLT?

There is a lot of crossover between PDT & CLT. CLT was a name coined by Bill Porter of CLT Clinics to represent the new generation of PDT treatment. Legally though, even though the acronym CLT has entered into popular language as a treatment description, only CLT Clinics (because they have registered the name) are officially authorized to use the term in a business context. There are however, quite a few clinics offering CLT type treatment—and so our question needs to be expanded to: apart from the second-generation photosensitisers, what are the other differences between conventional PDT and CLT type treatment?

Before CLT (and the associated development of new photosensitive agents) the focus of treatment tended to be just on the cancer tumour (in the same way that radiotherapy treatment is often focused upon a tumour and its immediate surrounding area). However, the new agents have opened up the possibility of treating an individuals whole body, with the aim of killing all cancer cells present—within the primary tumour, secondary metastasises and any free floating cancer cells in the bloodstream. This is done by irradiating an individual's whole body with the correct frequency of light, usually in the infrared range. This is achieved by positioning a number of correctly tuned light panels around the body. CLT Clinics have improved on this slightly, and are utilising a 'light bed' which more evenly irradiates the body with light.

Another design of recently developed PDT type treatments is that after an initial clinic visit, therapy can be carried out at home (using an agent plus an appropriate light source) over an extended period of time (rather than just one or two treatments at a clinic). This means treatment can adopt a more gentle and gradual approach—and while treatment progresses, focus can also be directed at building immune system health and strength. (Important note: a recent study found that Radachlorin agent was toxic when used orally on a daily basis, long term—more details later).

Ralph Moss's study and other controversial issues

The issues surrounding PDT and CLT are quite complex and involved, but they are important for you to appreciate (so as you can use your budget wisely). Therefore, we will spend some time looking at the most important details of the current controversy so to provide you with an independent and accurate description of events.

Until the fall of 2002, very few people in the alternative cancer sphere had heard of PDT. Around this time cancer treatment investigator Ralph Moss (see p.167 and p.5) mailed out a newsletter detailing some spectacular recoveries from cancer that were reputedly being obtained by CLT Clinics of Ireland. Many people—clinics, practitioners and those with cancer were excited by what they read and events after this date moved quickly. (As mentioned earlier, prior to this date, PDT was very much a proven therapy but was restricted to certain cancers and only available in specialised medical centres. Generally speaking most treatment was research based rather than clinically based. You can get a feel for the in-depth work that is being done in these centres by searching the PubMed database for the phrase PDT at: www.ncbi.nlm.nih.gov.) You will also find a document summarising many of these studies at the book linked website www.healing-cancer.co.uk/resources.

One of the first things that happened after Moss's newsletter announcement about CLT treatment, was that other clinics looked to source the same photo-sensitive agent that CLT Clinics was using—so that they could offer their patients this unique treatment as well. The agent CLT clinics were using at this time is called Radachlorin, developed by Andrei Reshetnickov in 1994, and now produced by a Russian company called Radapharma. Radachlorin is an agent made from spirulina. At the time we are discussing, CLT Clinics had struck up an exclusive business agreement with Radapharma for distribution of Radachlorin and so were in control of the agent and its availability. This agreement has now lapsed and so the field is now more open for Radachlorin. Some other clinics do now source the Radachlorin from Radapharma direct, while other clinics have begun to synthesise their own agent directly from spirulina.

CLT Clinics charged a considerable amount for treatment with Radachlorin agent. This caused CLT Clinics some subsequent problems, mainly in the form of some very dissatisfied CLT Clinic clients—because after CLT Clinics exclusive agreement with Radapharma lapsed, the same clients found out they could have purchased the same agent used by CLT Clinics for a substantially lower cost—though we should note that for proper treatment they would still have needed access to an infrared laser or LED panels.

After Moss, had announced the treatment being offered by CLT Clinics, he was contracted (by CLT Clinics) to carry out a study of patients they were treating. The study would focus on treatment, the period following treatment and outcome of treatment (after a minimum of six months) of forty-eight patients.

Moss's study was published in the December 2003 issue of Integrative Cancer Therapies (available from www.sagepub.com). However, during the study, Moss and CLT Clinics experienced some major difference of opinion about how treatment was progressing. The main reason, (in our opinion), on Moss's side, seems to have been that he was very dissatisfied, as well as frustrated, with the low level of therapeutic follow-up being offered by CLT Clinics in terms of basic patient care and CLT Clinic's seeming lack of interest in monitoring actual patient experiences and therapeutic outcome. This contributed to Moss, (in our opinion again), feeling that his relations with CLT Clinics needed more distance, so as to ensure the focus of the study remained firmly and squarely on patients and their direct experience of CLT, as well as to ensure the independence and integrity of the study.

The forty-eight patients in Moss's study were given the following CLT protocol:

1 Patients received Radachlorin photosensitising agent.

2 At the CLT clinic, the agent was initially intravenously injected (rather than given orally). Intravenous and corresponding light treatment was carried out repeatedly over a few days.

3 Agent illumination was carried out with a number of LED panels (tuned to the correct wavelength of light) sited around each patient's body.

4 After clinic treatment, patients continued treatment at home, for several months, taking Radachlorin orally.

5 Patients illuminated their bodies at home with infrared lamps (i.e. standard Philips Infraphil type lights). These emit a much broader spectrum of light, but do cover the wavelength needed to activate Radachlorin.

Unfortunately, in Moss's own words, 'CLT, in this group, was a qualified failure'[41] The abstract of Moss's reads:

'Cytoluminescent Therapy® (CLT) is an unconventional form of photodynamic therapy (PDT), utilizing a second-generation chlorophyll-derived photosensitizing agent and whole-body illumination. Starting in late 2002, CLT was administered in Ireland to 48 patients. Illumination with lasers and light-emitting diodes followed the administration of an initial bolus IV. After returning home, patients continued self-administered treatment using oral agent activated by infrared lamps. CLT proponents claimed that these procedures were beneficial to patients with advanced cancer. An organization devoted to making information on alternative therapies available to the public was engaged to contact these CLT patients and assess the outcome. In informal contacts, patients reported that initial side effects were generally mild and transient. However, especially after commencing self-treatment, many reported unanticipated effects, including fatigue and general weakness, increased pain, cough, dyspnea, diminished appetite and weight loss, tissue necrosis, and other major symptoms. At a minimum of 6 months after initial CLT, no patient has reported an objective response, and some have complained of deterioration on the home treatment. There have been 17 deaths among the 48, with a mean survival after initial treatment among decedents of 4.2 months. CLT, in this group, was a qualified failure, with a high incidence of after-effects. The mode of action of these after-effects has yet to be explored...'[42]

These findings came as a surprise (as they are in complete contrast with the positive treatment outcome descriptions Moss provided in his newsletter of the previous year). There are however, some observations in the study that need further clarification. For instance, treatment was carried out in four separate groups 1, 2, 3, 4 but when the groups are combined into two sets there are some startling but unexplained differences. For example, the mortality rate after six months in groups 1 and 2 combined was 54.2%, whereas groups 3 and 4 combined was 12.5%. Moss is not sure of the reasons for this difference, especially considering the fact that the number of stage IV malignancies treated was higher in groups 3 and 4: 70.8% for groups 1 and 2, and 79.2% for groups 3 and 4. Moss does mention some other factors that might have played an important role. Whereas for groups 1 and 2 no selection criteria were used in terms of who was accepted for treatment, groups 3 and 4 specifically excluded individuals who were:

'...bedridden, non-ambulatory, or confined to wheelchairs; who were receiving supplemental oxygen most or all of the time and were too sick to travel; who were suffering from severe cachexia; who had stents implanted for pancreatic or bile duct cancer; whose tumours comprised a major blood vessel or involved the spinal column; who were suffering from porphyria; who were clinically depressed and therefore unlikely to comply with treatment; who were younger than the age of 18; or who were pregnant or contemplated getting pregnant within 1 year of undergoing treatment'[43]

Further groups 1 and 2 (in contrast to groups 3 and 4) received other complementary cancer treatments along with the CLT treatment. These mainly consisted of:[44]

- Intravenous vitamin C, glutathione, AF2 (an liver and spleen extract from sheep), and sodium bicarbonate
- Complex homeopathic medications
- Intramuscular injections of thymus extract
- Ozone and oxygenation therapies

The fact that individuals in the first two groups (who did less well) received the above treatments as well as CLT raises the question as to whether the complementary treatments interfered and/or degraded CLT therapy. We asked CLT Clinics to provide their view as to what additional factors might have contributed to the different outcomes between the groups $1+2$ and $3+4$. Reasons they provided are as follows:[45]

- The main difference was the uncontrolled pain, inflammatory processes (not controlled in the first two groups).

- A significant number of individuals in the first two groups contracted flu while receiving treatment at the CLT clinic. Many of the patients seemed to be affected in their breathing (even though their lungs were not directly involved in the illness).

- The health of individuals in the third and forth groups were more stable.

- One patient's husband (from groups $1+2$) even brewed up a batch of his own photosensitiser and was dispensing it to some of the group.

More about CLT Clinics

As mentioned above, CLT Clinics have been subject to a lot of criticism over the last year; from clients who feel they were charged too much for the treatment, from clients who feel they didn't receive enough aftercare and support; and the severe criticism contained or at least implied in Moss's study. Our hope is that CLT Clinics have taken the criticism on board and have made improvements to the way they are operating.

Important note: Because CLT is far more expensive than many other therapies, and relationships between CLT Clinics and some of its clients have been very strained in the past, we recommend you clearly establish exactly what therapies you will receive; how they will be administered; how long the CLT photosensitising agent will be made available to you after you return home and what the procedure and costs will be of any repeat treatments needed. Further, and most important, how much of a say you will have in terms of obtaining repeat treatments and additional agent. Our hope is that CLT Clinics are now in a position to offer a long term relationship with their clients, rather than just a one off treatment, but for your own assurance and peace of mind you should ensure and take responsibility to ensure all these issues are addressed in their CLT Clinics written contract. We feel it is important for you to appreciate, that in terms of PDT/CLT type treatments becoming available to the public, that compared, say to the treatment of Dr Lechin, which has been established for many years and is supported by many professionally conducted studies, that

Agent by	Strength	Recommended Protocol	Toxicity	Cost
Seaweed based agent by CLT Clinics	Likely to be the highest strength agent	Taken orally. First treatment on light bed. Normal daylight levels considered sufficient to activate take-home agent	Reported to be low	€20,000 ($24,679) for light bed treatment and take home agent
Radachlorin (Radapharma spirulina extract)	Shown to exert significant effects against certain cancers.	Intravenous only for a limited number of treatments. Noted as toxic when taken orally for prolonged periods	Acceptable if used according to Radapharma guidelines	Different clinics offer different prices. Costs vary between €6000–10,000 ($7400–$12340)
Photostim (Radapharma)	Not ascertainable	Oral. Can be used with light source from either Radapharma or Operation Hope Clinic	Low	€250 ($308) for 100ml (lasts between 7–40 days depending on dose taken)
Operation Hope Clinic (AusChlorin)	Reported to be similar to Radachlorin	Always taken orally	Reported as low if used at recommended dosage	Approx €60 ($74) per week. Special wavelength light source costs €613

Table 10: Comparison of publicly available PDT/CLT agents

PDT/CLT treatments based on the newer agents are very much in the process of being worked out and hence should be termed experimental.

A more advanced agent than Radachlorin

Another fact needed to complete this complex picture, is that though PDT/CLT type agents are available through several sources, at the present time CLT Clinics agent appears to be the most powerful, and the least toxic. Though as an organization they charged (and still charge) considerably more than most other clinics are now charging for their own agent/treatment, we should note that CLT Clinics claim to have developed a more powerful and substantially less toxic agent than Radachlorin, as well as a special light bed (that completely surrounds the person being treated with the correct wavelength of light).[46] Most commentators still mistakenly believe that CLT Clinics are using Radachlorin as their photosensitising agent. However, no formal studies have yet been carried out to show that CLT Clinics new agent actually works better in the body than Radachlorin—at the present time, reports are only anecdotal.

One of the findings in the Moss study was that Radachlorin agent taken orally for a prolonged period produces toxicity problems. The manufacturers guidance is that it should only be used intravenously for a short period of time (please note: Radapharma now offer a less toxic agent for oral use called Photostim). However, CLT Clinics assert that taking their photosensitising agent *orally* (daily) over a four month period, is both simpler and more effective, and most importantly, that it leads to the agent being taken up in a way that delineates, far more clearly and finely, the boundary between the cancer and surrounding tissue (i.e. there is not so much spillover of agent from cancerous cells into surrounding healthy cells). CLT Clinics assert that there are no toxicity issues with their new seaweed based agent—and that they have completed laboratory toxicity studies documenting this.[47]

It appears that over the last two years, CLT Clinics have been developing an agent from photosynthetic bacteria (found in seaweed). Because seaweed grows underwater, often in shade, it is far more efficient at harvesting light then spirulina (which floats on the surface of water). CLT Clinics estimate their new agent is some two to three hundred times more powerful than Radachlorin— and as mentioned, assert it is significantly less toxic than Radachlorin. After the initial light bed treatment at their clinic, sunlight alone is considered sufficient to activate the take-home medication (i.e. no infrared light source is needed as was the case with Radachlorin).

In summary, we can note that PDT/CLT is an extremely significant treatment, even if it hasn't yet come of age. If you are considering the treatment, there are a variety of agents to choose from, (i.e. agents from different manufacturers, clinics and practitioners). Your choice will most likely be decided by the budget you have available. Table 10 below summarises the important facts about each agent. (Note: the majority of this table has been compiled from our own impressions, rather than from studies.)

Latest news

From reports appearing in Irish newspapers during May 2004, it is not clear how much longer CLT Clinics will be allowed to operate in Ireland itself.[48] However, we have heard that CLT Clinics is aiming to license clinics to use their new agent in various locations around the world, including the UK. (Contact CLT Clinics to find out clinics offering treatment with CLT agent.) Our view is that this is welcome news because clinics who maintain high standards of practice, ongoing client care and scrupulous follow-up will be able to use the agent in a way most beneficial for individuals with cancer. Please check out www.healing-cancer.co.uk for an update.

Contact details for agent manufacturers and clinics

With some of the contacts listed below it will be obvious which agent they are using for treatment. For others you may wish to enquire as the field is in flux and practitioners are changing agents frequently.

Radapharma public sales:

www.bioresource.biz/
client@bioresource.biz
Elan Group S.A.
Post address: 1108 Budapest, Agyagfejto ut.4, IX/36, Hungary
☎: +36 20 921 9017

Radapharma main site:

http://www.radapharma.ru

CLT Clinics Ltd.
PO Box 618
Killaloe
Co. Clare
Republic of Ireland

Shannon Airport is close by.

☎: 00 353 61 375815
🖨: 00 353 61 374910
E-mail: cltclinics@eircom.net
Website: www.cancerclt.com

The Dove Clinic for Integrated Medicine
Hockley Mill Stables
Twyford
Hampshire
S021 1NT
☎: 01962 718000, 🖨: 01962 718011

The Dove Clinic also offer several other treatments including immunotherapy and ozone therapy. PDT treatment costs approximately £8500 ($15745).

Latest News: At the time of going to press, news has it that The Dove Clinic is to begin offering PDT treatment with CLT agent rather than with other PDT agents. See healing-cancer.co.uk for confirmation.

Operation Hope Clinic (Run by: Professor Noel Campbell) – Offers clinic based treatment as well as agent and light sales to the general public.

Operation Hope Clinic utilise an agent similar to Radachlorin, and for take home use, the agent is taken orally. However, the agent is not taken daily, but rather a full dose is taken between one to three times a week. Taken this way seems to get around the toxicity problems reported in Moss's report.

Clinic: Level 5 167 Collins Street Melbourne Victoria Australia
Correspondence: Post Office Box 137 Parkville VIC 3052 Australia

☎: 03 9639 6090 International 613 9639 6090
🖷: 03 9639 4006 International 613 9639 4006
☎: (Prof. Campbell 0412 994 001 International 61412 994 001)
Email noelc@smile.org.au
Web www.smile.org.au

At the time of writing the IAT Clinic in the Bahamas (see p.134 for details) are intending to offer some form of PDT treatment in the near future.

IAT (Bahamas) Ltd.
P.O. Box F-42689
Freeport
Grand Bahama
Bahamas
☎: (242) 352-7455
🖷: (242) 352-3201

Email: burtonh101@aol.com
Web: www.iatclinic.com

Interview With Bill Porter (PDT/CLT)

Bill Porter is the founder of CLT Clinics. He became interested in the possibilities offered by PDT/CLT, after his wife Maggie contracted breast cancer. At the time the interview was carried out, CLT Clinics were using several protocols and methods that they have since changed (as described in the previous section). Of particular importance are the following:

- CLT Clinics were still in the process of developing their own seaweed based photodynamic agent, and so a fair amount of the discussion focuses on the spirulina derived agent in use at the time.

- Agent was being administered intravenously rather than by the present oral route of administration.

- Body illumination at the clinic was being carried out with LED panels rather than their recently developed light bed.

- Patients were being recommended to use infrared lights at home (to activate their take home agent), whereas now, normal daylight levels of sunlight are considered sufficient.

SK: Bill, to start with, before you describe the new generation of photodynamic agents you are presently working with, I'm wondering if you can say a little about previous photodynamic agents—the ones that have existed up until now?

BP: Well, the first agent that was widely approved is an agent called Photofrin. Photofrin is a mixture of derivatives from blood—usually pig's blood.

The properties of this material are that it selectively attaches to tumour cells compared to normal cells. The other property that it has in common with many types of *porphyrin* compounds is that it is photosensitive—which means that it absorbs energy at certain wavelengths of light.

When porphyrins absorb energy, the molecules become excited and their electrons shift to a higher level. In this state the molecules are unstable—and they therefore try to get rid of this instability. They do this by giving off energy in the form of electrons—i.e. they hand over free electrons to any oxygen that is in the surrounding area. It creates what is known as 'singlet oxygen'.

SK: Your describing that as porphyrin compounds become excited by certain wavelengths of light, they also become unstable and, in turn, get rid of this instability by donating an electron to another molecule. In practice you are saying that it is oxygen molecules that accept these electrons—and that this causes them in turn to become singlet oxygen—a highly unstable free radical.

BP: …extremely unstable… singlet oxygen oxidises any structures in its vicinity—though this action happens within a very small radius of effect and is very short-lived.

SK: I am wondering if the power of the singlet oxygen, in this case, comes from the fact that it's already inside the cell.

BP: Exactly, whatever it's around it will oxidise.

But different photo-synthesisers are more or less selective in their accumulation in cancer cells than others. For instance, Photofrin might typically have a selectivity of maybe one to three—which means that for every molecule that is injected intravenously, that maybe one will collect in a normal cell, and maybe three will collect in an abnormal cell like cancer.

But the compound we're using is collecting in, maybe, ten times that concentration—we're talking maybe one in thirty-five. Thirty-five times more might accumulate in a tumour cell compared with a normal cell.

SK: The compound you are engineering gets taken up by cancer cells far more readily than earlier agents?

BP: Very selectively and very preferentially.

SK: What is that process of it being 'taken up'? Why should a compound be taken up preferentially by cancer cells?

BP: It has to do with the fundamental difference between the metabolism of a cancer cell compared with a normal cell. The cancer cell, as we all know, has uncontrolled growth—it grows and compresses surrounding structures. In many cases it also has a corrosive effect on the surrounding structures.

One of the ways that cancer cells are able to do this is that they are not dependent on oxygen in the way normal cells are. In the normal structure of the body, each cell is fairly close to a little capillary that brings oxygen to it.

But cancer cells don't necessarily depend on oxygen carrying capillaries and their metabolism is an anaerobic form based on lactic acid.

SK: In the cancer cell, cellular respiration gives way to a fermentation mechanism—as Otto Warburg described. (See p.238 for details of Warburg's theory.)

BP: Correct. The other thing that's typical of tumour cells is that they have an extremely high rate of metabolism. They're taking in sugars at an extreme rate compared to normal cells—because they are growing and dividing [quickly]. So one of the things they do is to [virtually] monopolise the sugars in the body.

You can see this because people who have cancer can be wasting away elsewhere on their body, while the cancer tumour itself is growing phenomenally. The question though, is, what is it about the agent we are using that causes it to collect in those tumour cells?

The first thing is that the agent is slightly lipophilic, around 1:1.4

SK: Can you explain what this means?

BP: Lipophilic means that the agent is attracted to oily substances slightly more than watery substances. Now the way that sugars get into cells, is that they don't go directly in—rather they are carried in on what are called lipoproteins.

We could say that these lipoproteins are like horses on which the sugars catch a ride and are carried through the cell membrane into the inside of the cell. When they are through the cell membrane the sugars dismount and detach from the lipoprotein. The lipoprotein then goes back outside the cell into the blood stream to see if there's any more sugar available. If so, then they'll pick up any that are available and repeat the process.

Cancer cells are performing this process of bringing in sugars at an extremely accelerated rate. So when we infuse this molecule—our agent— into the bloodstream, they attach themselves to these lipoproteins and are carried inside the cell—almost like a Trojan horse. They're not sugars, but because they attach themselves to the lipoproteins they are carried inside the cell, and when inside, detach themselves.

The other thing that it does over time is to insinuate and intercalate itself into the DNA—and as it gets intertwined in the DNA it acts like a monkey wrench thrown into the DNA replication machinery.

SK: As you said—it's a real Trojan horse.

BP: Yes, it rides right along in with the lipoprotein. Cells have intelligence and defence mechanisms, and ways of living and surviving—but the nice thing about this compound that we're using is that it's almost like candy to a cancer cell. It goes right in—it's not seen as a toxic or offending substance the way a lot of the chemotherapy agents are. With most of the chemotherapy agents, after a while a huge resistance builds up.

SK: You mean that a cells' natural intelligence learns to keep the chemotherapeutic compounds out—so in the end they end up having no therapeutic effect for a person?

BP: Correct—it's almost like a resistance to antibiotics. You can kill off all the bacteria that aren't resistant, but maybe there are certain ones that are resistant—and they multiply rapidly and pretty soon all the germs are resistant. A similar process might be applicable for tumour cells in regard to chemotherapeutic agents.

But the nice thing about the agent we're using is that there's no resistance that builds up to it. It's never really seen as a toxic agent—so even if you're administering it to a person and after therapy there's some left (maybe because it hasn't been irradiated with enough light), resistance won't build up to it over time.

SK: It sounds as if you are using an almost flawless agent. Even if we sat down to design an agent along perfect lines—it would be very much along the lines you are describing.

BP: That's right.

SK: I have read that the agent is based on spirulina—a blue green algae commonly available from health shops. Compared with normal chemotherapeutic compounds it sounds so harmless and the last thing likely to be the source of a major cancer therapy—(though of course it is definitely a health promoting substance in naturopathic terms).

BP: I would say that we're discovering things that have existed throughout the ages. The reason I say this is that if we start examining what it is about this agent that makes it so valuable—then I would say that what we're really discovering is not something new, but something that is as ancient as life itself.

It is a long story, but in essence, the basic ring structure of porphyrins is present in all our bodies. If somebody has a tumour—say a lung tumour—then, before they've had any treatment for it, if you put a bronchoscope down into their lung and shine light of a certain frequency on the tumour, you would see it glowing—it would fluoresce under the right conditions.

SK: Those are the natural porphyrins fluorescing?

BP: Yes—because porphyrins have travelled around the body and selectively attached to the tumour. Obviously in this example the tumour is deep in the body and depending upon the type of porphyrin, it may be that not enough light has reached the area to kill the tumour.

But I am sure that in terms of other areas of the body, porphyrins acting in conjunction with sunlight function as a natural photodynamic therapy (PDT). Further, I am sure that it represents a major factor in our ability to rid ourselves of abnormal cells.

SK: Maybe I can ask you to describe, in a little more detail, about porphyrins. Is it the name of a certain chemical structure?

BP: Porphyrins are a class of compounds that have a so-called tetrapyrrole ring structure. In the liver (which is the major chemical factory of the body), carbon chains are stuck together to form something called aminolevulinic acid, ALA for short. If you take four or five of these ALA compounded chains and stick them together, then you get a five-sided circular ring. It is this ring that goes on to make haemoglobin—a similar process is used to make chlorophyll in plants.

SK: I am reminded that there is a remarkable similarity between chlorophyll and haemoglobin. Diagrammatically speaking, when the two chemical structures are placed side by side they are nearly identical, apart from the fact that haemoglobin has an iron molecule at its centre and chlorophyll has magnesium molecule. It's quite remarkable—chlorophyll is the direct equivalent of blood.

BP: Exactly—they're both intricately connected with effecting oxygen. As you know, chlorophyll is basically a harvester of energy and the agent we're using is a harvester of energy—it's derived from chlorophyll.

In plants, sunlight energises the chlorophyll. That energy is then used to split off the carbon from carbon dioxide. The carbon is then used to make cellulose [the building block of plants]. Carbon dioxide is composed of one carbon molecule and two oxygen molecules. As a result of this energy harvesting, O^2 is created as a by-product.

But you see, in the process that we're using for cancer, the agent harvests the light that we shine on it, but a different type of oxygen is created—i.e. O^1 – singlet oxygen. So the plants process, and the process we are using are analogous—that is, they are both harvesters of oxygen.

The same thing occurs within haemoglobin. As blood circulates it goes through the lungs and picks up oxygen molecules, which it then carries around the body. At the appropriate time, it sheds its oxygen as part of a chemical process to supply oxygen to our bodies.

SK: You're describing that you're tapping into a natural process—a process that is, literally, at the very heart of nature?

BP: Exactly.

SK: That makes me wonder, 'what could be responsible for this huge increase in cancer that has taken place in recent decades?' Is that a question you've asked yourself, and are green algae substances that are vitally important for correct body functioning?

BP: Walk down Oxford Street or Regent Street in London, and look at the fast-food restaurants and the massive amounts of food that are being consumed. How many green and yellow vegetables are being eaten? It's hardly any—it's mainly deep-fried hamburgers, pints of beer and sugary soda.

You see, it all fits, because there are certain cultures that don't suffer any cancer, or at least, they have very low cancer rates. However, people in these cultures consume large amounts of green substances that contain available chlorophyll. In addition, people in these cultures tend to get a lot of sunlight.

SK: I'm reminded that there is a specific 'school' of cancer based on the consumption of barley grass—The Hippocrates Health Institute founded by Ann Wigmore.[49] I have heard mixed reports about this particular therapeutic approach.

BP: But you see—they're only focusing on cancer treatment using massive amounts of chlorophyll. If you carry out the therapy in London, in December, then it's only going to have a limited effect compared to somebody who does it in Mexico or the Bahamas [unless you use a more active form of chlorophyll that is activated by lower ambient daylight conditions such as that found in seaweed].

SK: The value of sunlight to health is a huge issue these days. The general advice seems to be to block it out with sun creams.

BP: Well ultraviolet wavelengths at least. One major factor in this whole dynamic is that sunlight is a mixture of wavelengths of light. Sunlight goes all the way from extremely powerful but short wave length radiation, through to very long wave radiation.

Ultraviolet light (i.e. short wavelengths of light) is extremely intense, but the shorter the wavelength of light, the less it penetrates through tissue. So UV does damage the skin and cause skin cancer, but this is a separate issue from the longer wavelengths that penetrate into the body far deeper. Obviously if you go out into sunlight it doesn't burn your heart, even though it can burn your skin.

With regard to our treatment and skin cancer, we have seen excellent results if we put some of the agent that we are using on the skin and then shine a blue light on it (i.e. towards the 'shorter' UV wavelength end of the light spectrum).

But you see, it wouldn't help anything deeper if we put the agent on the skin in the same way. But if we introduce it internally, it turns out that there's a peak in the longer wavelengths of light that we can use. If we shine a long wavelength light that's tuned to a molecule that absorbs at that level, then even if the agent is attached to a deep tumour, the light penetrates sufficiently to activate it and to achieve the desired response—which is to take care of the tumour.

The wavelength of light enters into the equation in a major fashion. The next big leap forward in photodynamic therapy is going to be based not on using chlorophyll, but on something called bacteriochlorophyll (a red type of chlorophyll). Obviously plants that are used to being out in the light don't do as well if they are placed in the shade. Their chlorophyll is tuned to visual light. But there are other types of plants that have evolved with a type of chlorophyll that is extremely efficient at harvesting the higher wavelengths of light, even in the infrared range, for instance certain seaweeds.

A class of organisms called photosynthetic bacteria contain this bacterial chlorophyll. If you have an agent that is derived not from chlorophyll but from bacterial chlorophyll, and it's able to be activated in the infrared range (and everything else is nice with the agent in terms of being non-toxic, selective in terms of the cancer cells, and subject to rapid elimination), then you have the most ideal situation because you can treat the deepest tumours with great facility—because the infrared wavelengths of light travel deep into the body with ease.

Photosynthetic bacteria derived agents are going to be the next significant advance in CLT. What we have now seems to be working quite favourably, but it's only the beginning—only the beginning of the possibilities for this type of therapy.

SK: Your describing that agents based on photosynthetic bacteria found for instance, in seaweed, will work even better as a photodynamic agent because they are able to pick up infrared wavelengths of light far more efficiently than the chlorophyll compounds found in spirulina—and that this is especially important in terms of tumours that are located deep in the body.

BP: That's correct. I am thinking that I never got to fully answer the question you raised earlier about advantages of one agent over another. This seems to be a good time.

The original agents have a number of characteristics. Firstly, they weren't consistent in their quality, even from one batch to the next. In addition, with Photofrin (one of the early photodynamic agents), after it had been injected in an individual you'd have to wait two days before everything circulated round and had got to the point where it attached well enough to the tumour compared to normal tissue. However, with another agent called Phoscan, which is approved in the UK for treating head and neck cancer, you have to wait four days.

SK: And even then you're saying, it's not clear how preferentially tumour cells have taken up these early agents.

BP: Well, it's not nearly as preferential as you would like. The other factor is that after therapy has finished; the agents are not rapidly eliminated from the body. This means that patients have to cover up all exposed skin surfaces for a month after treatment because the slightest bit of sun exposure would give them a terrible burn. This can be the case with Photofrin and to a slightly lesser extent with Phoscan—and obviously this is not an ideal situation.

With our agent we only have to wait three hours after infusion before treatment can begin. Another advantage of our agent is that by the next day, essentially, it has been eliminated from the skin—so there's virtually no photosensitivity to sunlight.

SK: Can we go through the process that takes place when a patient visits your clinic?

BP: What we've been doing is that [after patients have arrived and settled in], we infuse the agent by intravenous infusion and then wait three hours— then we start doing the main part of the treatment.

We irradiate the area (containing the cancer) with light energy of the correct wavelength for the photodynamic agent we are using. This causes the chain reaction creation of singlet oxygen that goes on to kill the tumour.

SK: I understand you irradiate a person's whole body with the light (to wipe up stray cancer cells) rather than just focusing on the areas where you know tumours are present?

BP: Traditionally, with photodynamic therapy, most doctors treated the discrete tumour, for instance, endoscopically in the bronchi, in the oesophagus, or the bladder. They would irradiate just the single area.

That's fine if you just have one tumour—but as we all know, the main problem with tumours is that they metastasise—a little bit breaks off and then spreads throughout the body. In contrast, we've adopted a new approach, and that's why we've more or less shifted away from calling it photodynamic therapy, and are calling it Cellular Light Therapy or Cyto-luminescent Therapy.

It's a major shift away from localised treatment to systemic treatment.

SK: I am wondering about the following: let's say that ninety-five percent of a tumour has been killed by CLT treatment. What happens to the last five percent—does it tend to die off on its own later, because its larger structure has been compromised—or is it a case that you really have to kill every single cancer cell with the therapy?

BP: In addition to the cytotoxic effect from the light and the CLT agent, there are two other factors that, to varying degrees, enter into the equation. The first factor is that the process tends to cause coagulation in the new blood vessels that are feeding the tumour.

SK: It cuts off their food supply?

BP: Yes—the blood circulation around the tumour seems to shut down. You can even see it sometimes because by the end of the treatment, there's a sort of a purplish discolouration of tumours that are near the skin. It starts turning dark where we've killed the tumour.

The second factor—and this is a greyish area, is that when there is this fragmentation of millions of tumour cells as a result of the treatment, phagocytes or scavenger cells start picking them up as they start flowing into the blood stream and lymph system.

What seems to happen is that, for the first time, fragments of tumour cells are presented to the immune system. The question we are asking is, to what extent does this process lead to an increased and more effective immune response being generated?

SK: You mean that even though up to this point the patient's immune system hasn't been responsive enough to kill the tumour, this sudden onslaught gives it a kick?

BP: It's a little different to that. You see, the reason the immune system hasn't been killing the tumour is because tumour cells cloak themselves to avoid immune system recognition....

SK: But once cells start to break down, the immune system can get a hold on it—see it for what it is.

BP: It's my feeling that this is a factor that causes further response.

SK: I also understand that patients take some photosensitive agent home with them (along with an infrared light source)—so they can continue the therapy for the next few months?

BP: What we're trying to do is to carry on the same process on an ongoing basis—even when a person returns home. Fortunately, in the past several months, we have been able to formulate an oral form of the intravenous agent. Rather than just infusing it intravenously and giving the treatment here one time (even though it seems to have a massive effect on a tumour), I thought—why not keep hitting it at home on a daily basis?

Our patients take the oral agent for three to four months following the initial intensive treatment at our clinic.

I haven't mentioned one aspect of therapy, which I think is important to mention. Because these agents are extremely sensitive to light, it's possible, if treatment isn't done appropriately, that too much agent in combination with too much light could lead to a terrible photochemical burn on the skin. Our main thrust is to do no harm and one of the main things that we've done is to adjust the therapy so that we do not cause any of these photochemical burns.

SK: That sounds like an important factor that people need to bear in mind in deciding where and who they should receive the treatment from. I just want to thank you Bill, for everything you have explained to us.

BP: Thank you as well.

6

Interview with Ralph Moss

RALPH MOSS IS one of the world's leading authority's on conventional and unconventional cancer therapies. He has been deeply involved in the field for many years, and has played an important part in working to ensure unconventional cancer approaches are given a fair and realistic appraisal as to their merits. The large number of trials being conducted in the US at the present time—into the efficacy of many unconventional cancer treatments—are due, in no small part, to Dr Moss's persistence, patience and skills as a writer.

We hope that the following interview will bring you some of Dr Moss's expert knowledge. You can find more about Dr Moss's work at www.cancerdecisions.com

Interview With Ralph Moss (A Wider View Of Cancer Therapies)

Simon Kelly: Ralph, can we start with two of the therapies that we have placed in Group 3 of the table that forms the backbone of this book—Burton's Immuno-Augmentive Therapy (IAT) and Buzynski's Antineoplaston therapy.

Ralph Moss: Well, they're still on the scene. They've survived twenty to twenty-five years and they certainly can't be left out of any consideration. However, there hasn't been much activity around either of them in recent years, and I think that Burton's therapy deserves so much more of a serious investigation. But in both these cases there are political factors hampering their development—the antagonisms that were generated many years ago are hard to dispel in the present time, even though I don't think the same antagonisms that occurred then would occur today.

SK: Is that because the environment is much more receptive to alternative cancer treatments?

RM: No, I wouldn't say much more... But it is more receptive, and government officials in particular are on their best behaviour because there is congressional scrutiny now of any sort of malfeasances [wrong-doing by public officials] in regard to alternative cancer treatments. So the kind of high-handed activity that was absolutely the rule is not so possible now.

SK: You are referring to the maverick behaviour of the official cancer organisations and authorities?

RM: Well, I guess you could say maverick. I mean, they basically dealt contemptuously with all the would-be alternative treatments and were unrestrained in their arrogance. That started to come to an end in 1992.

SK: That was the year of the formation of the Office of Alternative Medicine...

RM: Yes, the Office of Alternative Medicine, now called the National Centre for Complimentary and Alternative Medicine (NCCAM). When this was formed it became impossible to blindly attack alternative methods without also simultaneously attacking a branch of the NIH (National Institutes of Health). This had repercussions and so only a very tiny minority of scientists and doctors kept up the attack in the original form.

However, there's a rearguard action, by the so called 'quackbusters', but it is very much rearguard and as they leave the scenes due to natural attrition I don't think we're going to see these kind of attacks continue.

I lived through some very heavy fighting that occurred around this and I think there's a tendency for it to start again if those words, those buzz words are mentioned. It starts to re-enflame the old antagonisms. We're not yet at the point where we can have a serious academic study of Burzynski, IAT or Laetrile. I cover most of this in 'The Cancer Industry'. It's still a little too hot.

SK: Yes, and it's interesting because over here in the UK there are not the same passions around alternative cancer treatments. In fact most people, including those in the medical profession, probably don't know about the existence of any of them.

RM: Right, they don't know about them. On my few visits to the UK I found if anything, that there was a more oppressive atmosphere. I don't think the alternative movement and practitioners in the UK have even got far enough in to represent a challenge. In the US, Laetrile was a tremendous challenge to orthodox medicine.

SK: Yes, over here in the UK there are very few doctors using the kind of treatments described in this book

Regarding challenges, what has been so long needed are properly run trials for alternative treatments. Thankfully, I note that the Office of Cancer Complementary and Alternative Medicine in the US are presently running a whole series of important studies. Looking through the list, there are trials on pancreatic enzymes, mistletoe lectin, shark cartilage and many others. Really, these are the sort of trials that proponents of alternative cancer therapies have been asking for, for many years?

RM: Definitely, and the pancreatic enzyme one is particularly important. But there are a lot of difficulties in arranging trials like these and I'm not sure that we have got to a point where the results will be accepted as a definitive truth, or even proof of principal of any of these treatments.

And I say this because of the fact that the pancreatic enzyme study was not able to be randomised. If and when that trial turns out positive, there will be howls of protest from medical journals and so forth, that it's not really a proper trial.

And there is no true randomisation in the trial. The reason being, that the patients themselves refused to go into a randomised trial. It is very important to understand that it wasn't possible to recruit people for the trial, who on the basis of randomisation [i.e. chance] would either receive a completely alternative treatment with [enzymes], coffee enemas and so forth—or chemotherapy.

Using an analogy, it's a bit like when World War Two broke out. If you pooled all the recruits and all the young men, and you said, 'Well, now we're going to randomly send you to the Nazi army or to the British army'. What kind of people would not know which side they were fighting for, or what side they wanted to be on?

It's a tremendous selection bias to say we're going to randomise and only have people who don't know the difference between chemotherapy and coffee enemas.

The public go straight to the internet and is so dichotomised that people more or less know whether they want to go with their orthodox oncologist and be offered a few months of extra survival—perhaps. (This is what is basically claimed for Gemsar, the standard drug for pancreatic cancer). Or—the possibility of a cure with a very non-conventional treatment. People know [about these choices] so by the time that they call about the trial they already more of less know that they want to go into the pancreatic enzyme study. If we tell them that we're going to choose for them, they back out. Maybe only one, two or four per cent of the patients agreed to be randomised, and I suspect the reason that they agreed to be randomised was that they knew that they could always pull out of the study if they found that they had got into the wrong arm of it.

SK: You mean—because individuals are able to work out which treatment they are receiving, if things seem to be going badly for them, then they will withdraw from the trial or swap over to the treatment the other group is receiving.

This critique of RCTs (Randomised Clinical Trials) is often voiced by practitioners in the alternative field. Their argument is that it's unethical to decide for individuals which treatment they should receive. A full-blown RCT study means half of the individuals taking part will not receive the newer potentially more beneficial treatment.

RCT's are a good idea on paper—but how relevant are they to patients?

RM: Of course, randomised clinical trials are a great concept. Hill came up with the concept of randomisation in the late 30's and it became the 'ethical' way of conducting studies in the 40's... I think we're at a point where we can say that the randomised trial is one of those ideas that are terrific in the abstract.

SK: A proper randomised clinical trial (RCT) or phase 3 trial seems to represent the pinnacle of scientific investigation, doesn't it?

RM: It does—and everybody preaches the gospel of RCT's (randomised controlled trials), but in practice they are extremely difficult to do because they are fraught with all kinds of ethical and methodological problems.

I have spent a lot of time looking at the basis for approval of chemotherapy drugs and also for the general view of radiation as a proven method of treating cancer. What I would say in general is that for the last twelve major chemotherapy drugs that have been approved by the Food and Drug Administration in the US, that they have not been approved based on phase three trials. They have been approved based on phase two trials.

SK: Phase two trials not being an RCT but rather a comparative trial between a new drug and an existing drug.

RM: Well, it's not a comparison at all. It's just basically giving the treatment and then studying the response rate—there is no comparison. You can only do a historical comparison, which is usually meaningless.

SK: You mean a phase two trial might enable us to say for instance that patients do better on a new drug than the old drug.

RM: Right—but then again you haven't controlled the very things that led to the creation of the randomised controlled trials, i.e. selection bias and other biases. For instance, you don't know if the patient's lived fourteen months with the old drug and now they're living sixteen months with the new drug—or what the selection criteria were.

Unless the study is done concurrently, in the same institutions, at the same time, using the same treatment, same methodologies and diagnostic procedures, there's a million ways that the results could diverge. The whole idea of the controlled trial is that you control the variables so you can really [compare the results] head to head.

That hasn't happened. Sometimes phase three trials might be done after the drug has been approved, but for the last twelve major drugs approval was based only on phase two trials—small studies of thirty or forty patients.

SK: It's such a small number of patients to approve a drug. I was shocked when I read about that in your book, Questioning Chemotherapy. Most people have the impression that chemotherapy drugs are based on studies involving thousands of people—not forty or fifty.

RM: That's right—there's more than a million new cancer patients a year in the US and proportional numbers in the UK. Six to nine million worldwide a year getting cancer. And from that you can only recruit thirty or forty people.

It shows you how desperate this whole situation is. It just doesn't correspond to the needs of the cancer patient who's in the last stages of trying to cope with this disease.

SK: Can you say a little more about chemotherapy, because it is a subject you have written so much about. There is often the suggestion in your writings that chemotherapy is not as effective as many people presume.

I hear you say this on the one hand, but then I often hear of people who have had success with it. For instance, I recently heard of someone who received chemotherapy for a tumour on their spine. They received chemotherapy for a short while and now the tumour seems to have gone. Someone else had a double mastectomy and chemotherapy and is fit and healthy over twenty years later.

It's very difficult to put what you have found through your research together with cases like these.

RM: Oh Absolutely. There are a few things at work here. One that you have to be conscious of is the post-hoc, ergo-procta-hoc fallacy. Just because they had a double mastectomy and chemo, and then didn't have a recurrence, doesn't mean it was the chemo that prevented it from happening.

In the case of breast cancer, stage one or even stage two, the majority of women, and in the case of stage one, the great majority, will not have a recurrence, and even if they do have a recurrence, will not die of their breast cancer, whether they have chemo or not.

Chemo is just the icing on the cake, and secondly, you can't argue, as Ulrich Abel said in 1990, for gambling based on the profits of the winner. Rather you have to look at the totality of what happens when people go through a particular regime because it's very possible that some people will benefit, maybe dramatically, while others will be harmed. Let's just say, that this woman had the chemo and it tracked the tumours on her spine. However, we don't know from that, how many other people might, to put it bluntly, have died from the chemotherapy or might have been crippled by the chemotherapy, or whatever. You always have to look to the totality of people treated rather than the person who benefits, who in fact might be the exception to the rule.

The third point I'd like to make is that it's possible. Chemotherapy is powerful and it can shrink tumours in cases like the above and for the case of tumours on the spine, it's probably a good idea to do it.

I'm not in any way arguing that one necessarily shouldn't [use chemotherapy]. However, as a general rule, what we need proof of is that shrinking tumours correlates with improved survival or prolonging quality of life.

In the case of a tumour on the spine, if a person has been crippled and can't move and can't walk, and then they give chemo and the person can then walk, I think there's a defacto assumption that this has improved their quality of life—although you'd have to ask [the particular individual] to find out if that's true—because one could easily conceive of a situation where a person could technically walk but was so sickened by the chemo that they felt their life wasn't worth living.

You have to really probe this scientifically and check that their life is improved by the treatment. Measurements of lifestyle and quality of life—they're tricky, because often, in my opinion, there is leading going on, leading questions on the questionnaires. Basically the doctors are skewing the questionnaire to get a positive answer.

You have to be very cautious about this, because if you asked other questions you might get an entirely different picture. The other point is… we do know that for the great majority of cancers, a partial response does not correlate with any increased survival (i.e. shrinking the tumour as opposed to obliterating the tumour)—though it can offer a wonderful sense of hope for the patient.

SK: Maybe, for the cancer patient, the first shrinkage never gets forgotten for the rest of the time they receive the treatment?

RM: Also, you could say 'well it offers hope and therefore it's a positive thing', but on the other hand we often hear the term 'false hope' banded about [in a negative way] against alternative treatments. Also, it could work both ways in that after you've had that shrinkage, then you find out that in fact it's back, that it's more aggressive.

In the long run, my opinion is that for the great majority of cancers a partial response does not mean anything in terms of survival, although it could mean something positive or negative for a person's quality of life.

Regarding 'complete responses'—there usually aren't enough of them to be able to make any statement about what effect the treatment has on survival.

Statistically, when you look at the aggregate group you find that for most kinds of cancer there isn't much of an argument to be made for chemotherapy if you're just talking about the standard measurements of benefit.

I think the benefits are mostly the feeling that you're dong something and the hope that you'll be one of the rare survivors. The commonsense [notion is] that by shrinking [the tumour], that you're doing something positive—though in fact you maybe doing something negative.

You may [in fact] be eliminating immune cells because the tumour is often made up of a cancerous core, surrounded by inflammatory tissue and also by a great many white blood cells. It's a bit like bombing a battle field where your own troops are surrounding the enemy.

SK: The white blood cells are keeping the cancer in check to a certain extent…

RM: Yes, exactly. Perhaps they are, they're certainly trying to. And you come in and you bomb the entire complex. You kill off a lot of the cancer cells and you kill off a lot of your own troops as well.

SK: I guess the rational is, 'OK, we're going to lose some of our own troops but at least we're going to get the whole lot in one go'. With radiation it often seems that the strike can be more precise—more of a clean surgical strike. Why doesn't that tend to work in practice?

RM: Well, I don't know why it doesn't work. There are two reasons that it might not. One is that it is likely that the cancer is more disseminated than we have given it credit for…

SK: You mean that cancer is a systemic illness—not a local one—i.e. that cancer is a general illness that over time becomes local—not a local condition that becomes general.

RM: Yes, I think there's a lot of merit to the idea that alternative doctors have [espoused] for a long time—that cancer is a systemic disease and that it arises from a problem in the body as a whole, the organism as a whole.

The notion of radiation is, of course [that it] is a local, regional treatment—the idea being, that the cancer spreads in an orderly fashion from a single cell outwards. So there is an emphasis on local regional treatment.

However, the more widespread use of chemotherapy, especially for breast cancer, was an acknowledgement by the orthodox medical community of these notions that had been kicking around in the non-conventional climate—that cancer from the [start] is really a systemic disease.

That's why they sometimes even give chemotherapy to stage one breast cancer patients—because we know it's around in the body.

SK: That's interesting—the point that chemotherapy is almost an acceptance of the idea that cancer is a systemic illness. But what about cancer—what really is it?

In this book we examine several different theories of cancer (see p.231 for details). Out of all of them, is there one you think is most likely to turn out to be the one that is true—or do you think all of them are true at different times?

RM: I do believe that the Trophoblastic theory is still the one to beat. I haven't seen anything that really refutes it. In fact, I think that with the development of stem cell science, we're approaching a kind of rapprochement between conventional science and the alternative world. Though I don't think that the conventional doctors are aware of the fact that they are treading on well-trodden ground when they talk about totipotent stem cells.

SK: Can you just elaborate on that a bit...?

RM: Well, I think that the notion of John Beard was that some germ cells get left behind in the process of embriogenesis [the formation and development of the embryo]. When triggered (though I don't believe that in Beard's days they knew what those triggers were) by what we would call an initiator or carcinogen, these left-over germ cells turn into or give rise to a kind of embryo, in the wrong time and wrong place.

[On the other hand] stem cell research is [also] saying that stem cells exist all over the body and they were left behind in the process of embriogenesis. [Further that] the purpose of them is that they initiate healing and re-growth [Beard didn't actually know what the germ cells outside of the gonads were for—but speculated that they were left over from embriogenesis]. So the term 'totally potent stem cell' and its concept is almost identical to what Beard talked about a hundred years ago.

I [think we can safely say that there are no] differences between them, even though the totally potent stem cell was 'discovered' and patented only five or six years ago. Already there's some work in the mid-west that is looking at the question of the transformation of these stem cells.

In other words, what happens when a stem cell itself becomes cancerous? They're already working in this direction and I think it's only a matter of time before someone is going to come up with the bright theory that cancers in fact arise not from the mutation of somatic cells, which has all kinds of philosophical difficulties of how something evolves backwards. But [rather and] much more logically, cancer would seem to arise from something that is moving forward evolutionary, but not getting very far and not getting all the way there.

I think it's just a matter of time before we hear that the cause of cancer is not somatic mutation, but the mutation of the stem cell. [Mutation of] the totally potent stem cell, by X-rays or chemical carcinogens or whatever triggers it off, sunlight, etc...

These cells are all over the body... They're left behind for a purpose [but] they can become cancerous...

SK: When you say, they are 'left behind', I am not sure what you mean—stem cells are just a part of all normal tissue aren't they?

RM: They are, yes. When I say left behind—I mean that in Beard's original conception (formed from watching the process in animals) germ cells migrate [to the gonads] in the process of the formation of the embryo. They have to get to their home, which is the gonads.

As this army of germ cells, (which is the future of the race, the future of the organism)—migrate through the developing embryo, some stragglers are left behind. These stragglers are deposited into different parts of the embryo, which then go on to become the organism.

So, you've got these little germ cells, not just in the testis or the ovaries, but all around the organism. Some day one of these might misfire and develop and try to make a little baby.

SK: Beard postulated a relationship between these germ cells, and enzymes being secreted by the pancreas—i.e. enzymes deactivate germ cells (in their trophoblast phase) and leave them vulnerable to destruction by our immune systems (see p.238 for more details of Beard's theory). Where are we in terms of either proving or disproving that linkage?

RM: I haven't seen that coming from the orthodox side yet. [However] I think that some bright person will either stumble across [Beard's] theory and become taken with it or else we'll have to reinvent the wheel.

Essentially [Beard] asked himself, 'what is it that stops the development of these trophoblasts?' And he knew from his work as an embryologist that the human embryo begins to produce [pancreatic enzymes] on the 56th day when there's no need for digestion.

SK: It's that linkage that really shows the importance of enzymes and why they are promoted so heavily in alternative cancer treatments.

RM: Unlike many things in alternative medicine, [the use of pancreatic enzymes] is not empirically derived. They really came out of this theory. It's a good theory.

SK: It was quite an insight by Beard

RM: It was tremendous, I mean it's just amazing to me that the world hasn't picked up on this and recognised how brilliant it is. Gonzalez in New York, with the group whom enzyme therapy is being tested on, is trying to demonstrate both the empirical value of the enzymes and also the validity of the theory.

If enzymes indeed do act, and pancreatic enzymes do have this anti-cancer activity—and I believe they do—then one would have to say, 'why do they do this and how in nature do they function?' We know that there is some evidence that enzymes do circulate in the body, in the bloodstream, and not just in the intestines.

SK: The Beardian theory is the one that you've really plumped for in your heart—in terms of the theory most likely to describe the process of cancer?

RM: Oh yes—in my heart—definitely. I recognise the difficulties in proving every aspect of this theory—but yes, that's what I believe. In fact this was the first theory I ever learned about cancer but I think it's stood up well and I hope and believe that the stem cell work will eventually converge with this Beardian theory.

[However] there are strong reasons not to acknowledge the early predecessors that have to do with patents and priority. You're much less of a genius if you've rediscovered the work of some obscure 19th century embryologist than if you come up with a new and original theory.

SK: Without being cynical, I suppose it's likely that the theory will be reinvented in a patentable form. With regard to the Beardian theory, I have read that you feel it is was a mistake of the Krebs's to link it with B-17 and Laetrile (see p.243 for details).

RM: Right, I think that it was a mistake. I don't think there was any inherent connection between Laetrile and Beard except that the same person [Krebs] was advocating them. [The result was that] it dragged the Beardian theory into the morass of Laetrile [politics], which was characterised by unscientific attitudes on both sides. It became a political battle rather than a scientific discussion. I don't know who is to blame.

SK: As you have mentioned Laetrile (B-17), I have noticed that to obtain anti-cancer action with Laetrile it is necessary to use extraordinary high levels of it—or at least that is what the animal studies show. I don't know how ascertainable the levels are for a person on a daily basis.

RM: You know—I lost my job at Kettering because of upholding the fact that Dr Sugiura had found that with a very high rate—a very high level of injected Laetrile—a definite anti-cancer activity [was observed]. Whether you could sustain that or reproduce that, I don't know. But I do feel that within certain limits, one has to be absolutely forthcoming to the public with scientific findings and not shape the findings to conform with your public relations needs.

That's what was happening at Kettering and I still feel it was unconscionable. I still think that there are some interesting things about laetrile, and some people are still looking at it. [In my opinion] neither the furious attacks against it, or the exaggerated claims made for it by some people were justified.

SK: Have any noteworthy findings about Laetrile been made or reported in recent years?

RM: No, I don't think so. There was a group in London at Imperial College who were working on a cyanide compound derived from another plant, cassava I think. It raised a lot of laughs because it was so obviously laetrile. It was interesting—but you know, most people are smart enough to stay away from something that's going to ruin their career.

SK: Personally I always consider it's a useful preventative.

RM: It's possible. I really wouldn't rule it out—but I just don't have any good evidence for that. It's really, at this point, sort of ancient history.

SK: I'm wondering if we can move on and cover some more of the big players in the alternative cancer field—for example, Naessens, Burton and Burzynski. Maybe you can give your impressions of them. Let's start with Burton—he always seems a brilliant but tragic figure.

RM: You know, I think that's true.

SK: Did you have occasion to meet him?

RM: Oh yes, a few times—I went down to his clinic four times. He was fascinating… and he was an amazing raconteur and… monologist. I once sat for hours and hours listening to him in force, and it was quite astonishing. [However] he could be very unpleasant… He was not a person who knew how to conduct himself in disagreements with people, yet he was always getting into disagreements and he had no skill in that department.

I think some of the problems with the NCI [National Cancer Institutes] were of his own making. Some of them wouldn't have happened to other people. He was the kind of person that once you'd crossed swords with him it was like he just created this desire [in you] to get even—to really let [him] have it.

I realised I felt it in myself and so I can understand how other people felt the same way. He was, literally, his own worst enemy.

His theory was close enough to conventional immunotherapy to be tantalising and different enough to raise the hackles of others in immunotherapy. He was not a major player in the immunology community—he was sort of jumping the line.

SK: An upstart, as you referred to him.

RM: Yes, he was an upstart, exactly.

SK: And what about his results?

RM: Well, it's hard to say, very hard.

SK: Have you kept an eye on people that have been to his clinic in the Bahamas over the years.

RM: You know—people who go to alternative clinics—many of their cases just don't constitute a reliable foundation on which to make claims for a treatment.

Oftentimes they have already tried other [treatments]—people might go for secondary prevention and yet they don't realise that's what it is. [For instance] they've been diagnosed, and their tumour has been removed. They might have a very high chance of a recurrence but they go [for the alternative treatment] and the tumour doesn't recur. If it does occur, well of course those people are not brought forward as examples. And the ones that don't recur—[well] you never know whether the cancer would have recurred anyway.

In recent years there's been a couple of attempts made to compile a best-case series [for IAT]. I've read both of those reports and looked at the cases and also I went down and looked at other cases about two years ago.

I'm convinced that in some instances treatment was effective and led to long-term survival. But again, we're not talking about very many cases and I don't know how those cases relate to the vast numbers of people who have received the treatment.

I would say, or the best I can say is, 'yes, it does work in some cases'. In addition, there is some evidence now, unpublished but scientific, that the treatment does enhance the immune system. I don't think it was classical quackery the way it was depicted—that was a very unfair characterisation [of IAT treatment] based in part on Burton's own personality and history.

SK: Burton's astounding demonstrations with the mice; were you able to observe them yourself?

RM: I never saw them—I saw the mice but I didn't see the actual disappearance of the tumours.

SK: Those demonstrations must rate as sone of the most noteworthy demonstrations in the history of science.

RM: Absolutely. Pat McGrady Sr who arranged [the demonstrations] for the American Cancer Society back in the 60's was a friend of mine. He was the science editor for the American Cancer Society and he and I talked about it and there was absolutely no question in his mind that they were genuine. Pat McGrady Sr was a very hardnosed reporter who knew his way around the block and wouldn't be taken in easily.

The explanation [given by mainstream critics] was that [the demonstrators] had massaged the tumours with their thumbs, liquefied them, and then extracted the liquefied tumour with a syringe.

I think it would take an enormous amount of nerve and skill to be able to pull something off like this—that's if it's even physically possible? I have no idea. This was the kind of crazy explanation I grew up with in order to avoid the obvious. They didn't want the credit for this to go to this upstart [Burton and his team]—and at the same time they were negotiating with them and various people in their labs. Sloan Kettering was trying to get them over as well.

SK: I'm remembering a line in your book—The Cancer Industry. It's a very memorable line—you indicate that Burton was intending to hand his findings over for nothing, and that Sloan Kettering had sent someone over to Burton's lab to investigate. You quote this investigator saying to Burton, 'if you're going hand your discovery over to us for nothing, it must be a load of crap'.

RM: Yes—a load of crap. Well, anyway that's Burton. IAT probably does have some validity to it. [In the future] the main interest would be to see if it does work—and why and where that happens.

Naessens does another [treatment]—I mean all of these people tend to be outsiders.

It's a kind of crazy field. Ordinary people become oncologists—everybody in this field is a bit different. Naessens is very different and I think with Naessens there are two aspects—one is the theory and one is the treatment. Again, as with Laetrile, I'm not sure I see the intrinsic connection between the two.

The theory is fascinating; I mean you just fall off your seat looking at it.

SK: Have you had a look down the somatoscope? (See p.80 for details.)

RM: I went four times. I kept going back, it really was amazing…

SK: Did you really feel that you saw something of the future—something that is true but is not at all known about or accepted in science?

RM: Exactly—it was like seeing a UFO. I mean how can these things be present in the blood—in your own blood, and yet no one ever told you about them? You can look through all the haematology textbooks and you won't find them. There's this whole system [of somatid's], this whole classification that Naessens has made—it's just mind-boggling.

And Naessens is very charismatic—so there's that. Now there are other people who are affiliated with more orthodox positions, who have belatedly said, 'yes, [these forms] do exist in the blood—however, they are…'—and then they enumerate different things that they could be. For instance they could be triglycerides or cholesterol, or a bit of fat popping around in the blood. There are some arguments that this is what the small somatids could be.

What you see [through the microscope] looks different depending on what meal [the patient] had that morning. But Naessens will tell you very confidently—'oh no, we know what the fat particles look like and they're different from the somatids'.

I'm not skilled enough to be able to differentiate. The bigger things that are floating around which he thinks are sort of expansions of the somatid cycle are sometimes described [from the orthodox point of view] as being the exterior membrane of red blood cells. [The theory being that] as they die and are destroyed, they kind of float away.

Whether this is a new science in the making or a pseudo-science, I don't know—but I do know that for a long time the medical establishment thought they could deal with him just by brushing [his work] aside.

However, a lot of lay people and some scientists have taken a look at [Naessens' discoveries] and said, 'we see something here'. And naturally your tendency is to accept the explanation of the discoverer.

As far as 714-X goes, I have no doubt that injecting a camphor product into the body, and presumably into the lymphatic system, will have some kind of profound effect—positive or negative.

I know it certainly seems to tune up the immune system, and has a psychological effect as well. But I've never seen any clear demonstration of any anti-cancer effect—at least in the people who are mostly stage four, terminal patients who take it. I don't think the cases that have been brought forward are [that] compelling. So, yes, I think it's some kind of bioactive substance, it has something. There's something there, but what it is, is something that should be studied a lot more. Again, it's a political hot potato, nobody really wants it, so we're sort of stuck in this case.

The third treatment you mentioned is Burzynski's. I do believe in his treatment. It's produced some wonderful results for a couple of kinds of cancer. He believes he has the answer to cancer—he thinks this is it. I have never heard him say otherwise. He's very brilliant and he's much better attuned to contemporary science than either Naessens or Burton was. He sometimes publishes and he is hooked into the clinical trial system through the FDA and so forth—he's a real fighter.

SK: From descriptions of the trials and difficulties Burzynski has endured over recent decades, I get the feeling he's a person who can really stand on the edge and see how far the institutions dare to push.

RM: That's right—he's an amazing guy. He's brave like the Polish people tend to be and very, very caring. But I have never been convinced that there's been good results in cancers other than lymphoma and brain cancer. So the battles have tended to be over the brain cancer cases and the people who believe in it, see a benefit, and those who don't—don't. It just seems to have got stuck—it doesn't seem to be any further along than it was three years ago.

SK: Can we turn to critics of alternative cancer approaches like Saul Green. He's so negative. I was just reading some of his writings again. It's quite a shock to read them especially as he writes in a very credible way. For instance he writes that no link between the immune system and cancer has ever been established.

RM: That's an extinct point, because you won't find that point of view in any text book on cancer today. I think it's to do with his own bitterness about not having been given what he thought was sufficient credit for various things.

SK: Would that have to do with the supposed similarity of tumour necrosis factor with Burton's IAT?

RM: Well, I think that's just part of it—he was part of the team that discovered tumour necrosis factor and perhaps there were some disagreements over that. He is somebody who I think is coming at this from the wrong direction.

SK: It's really difficult to relate to why he's so negative. It seems that he relegates anything apart from accepted conventional therapies into a category labelled, 'hippy-type spiritual namby-pamby crap'.

RM: He does have a psychological aversion to non-conventional treatments and I think the less I say about it, the better. My feeling about Saul Green is that he'll pass from the scene—it won't make much difference.

SK: Is his funding drying up now?

RM: I don't see much activity there and, you know—dogs bark but the caravan moves on.

It's no longer debatable whether or not alternative treatments are going to have a place in medicine—they have a place and it's just a question of where you draw the boundaries. Essentially the quackbusters lost the war—they just don't realise it yet.

As for the notion that the immune system has nothing to do with cancer. Look in any cancer textbook—it clearly has something to do with it. [However] I think it's true that it's not a one-to-one correspondence.

SK: The point of view from the quackbusters is that if you test the immune systems of cancer patients, they will come out normal…

RM: It's true, but they're tilting at windmills. They're tilting at the immune surveillance theory which was the first iteration of this relationship between the immune system [and cancer] by Thomas and Burnet in the 1950's.

SK: What are the newer theories about the immune system? I suppose that most of us only consider the immune surveillance theory—the idea that our immune system watches over our body for mutant cells.

RM: Right—but of course there is the question of the actual status of the immune system. Even though you're measuring numbers of cells, are those cells active or not? Naessens for instance can show you beautiful examples of white blood cells that are totally inactive.

SK: You're describing that its about the quality of the immune system, not just numbers of cells.

RM: Qualitative—exactly. The conventional tests only measure the quantita-
tive. In that sense I think that Saul Green performs a useful function if he
points out the deficiencies in some of the conceptions of cancer. But
there's an animus [i.e. prejudice] there that is hard to explain based just on
the science.

SK: One useful thing he does point out is that care needs to be taken when
making claims about a particular treatment. It's easy for a simple cause and
effect to be assumed between a treatment and a cure—when in fact there
could have been many other factors responsible for the healing.

RM: I think that is the question of the clinical trial.

A person like Saul Green—I've never seen him make any criticisms of
conventional medicine.

To me, that is a give-away, because if you are really concerned about
abuses—then what about the approval of chemotherapy based on phase
two trials? What about the lack of documentation of surgery and radiation
as proven therapy?

When you only criticise one side—and this has been said many times
about advocates of alternative therapy—it definitely gives the impression
that you are functioning on behalf of one side of an argument.

You're not really aiming at the truth—rather you're aiming at promoting
something. The only thing you accomplish by knocking the alternatives, (if
you don't concurrently point out the weaknesses of the other side)—is to
promote people going to the major cancer centres and just doing what
they are told by their oncologists.

SK: The bottom line is that we want to know the truth. It's not about taking
sides; it's about finding out the truth about these alternative therapies?

RM: Right. There is a lot of tendentious [i.e. biased] literature and as to what its
motives are—you'd have to ask the people who are writing it.

SK: So, working towards summarising all that we have spoken about—can I
ask you how many people you have provided your special reports for?

RM: I don't know—thousands.

SK: What's your kind of general advice to people when they come to you with
cancer?

RM: First of all, we try to see what benefit they could derive from the conventional treatments. It's important not to miss an opportunity just because
of a revulsion to the bad side effects of a treatment. You want to make sure

that where there is proof of an effectiveness of conventional treatment, that the person isn't over reacting and going headlong in the opposite direction.

SK: What would be some examples of these be?

RM: Surgery for stage one breast cancer; chemotherapy for testicular cancer; radiation for a variety of different cancers.

It's not always clear-cut, but my attitude is that people should do their best to get into the conventional literature. They should go to the US government's web site and look at the state of the art in terms of conventional treatment. People should make sure that they are getting state of the art [treatment]. Often I see people being recommended treatments, pet theories of different doctors that have no relationship to what is considered to be the standard treatment according to the US government.

The government maintains a very good website at cancer.gov, and people should familiarise themselves with that. Secondly, you want to know the credibility of the alternative practitioner—how long they've been in business, and how well founded the treatments that their using are. There's a wide variety in these treatments.

SK: How do you advise people—for instance do you say, 'Burzynski's would be a good way forward in your case'—or, do you make general health improvement recommendations?

RM: I use both. If I have some reason to believe that Burzynski has achieved good results in brain cancer, I will certainly tell people that. But I'm not the NIH, I can't do the best case series. It's hard enough for the NCI with its billions of dollars to carry out best-case series.

I look at cases and I visit. I'm trying to establish the credibility and the plausibility of the different treatments in different clinics. But you have to be modest in this because the hard work has to be done by the practitioners themselves and by the government.

It's a process I've been involved in for ten years at the governmental level and it's only now taking its first steps. I try to establish the viability of a clinic. It's also important to know how people are treated, because a lot of time some things look good on paper, but then you find in practice that they are a mess. It's just trying to find a happy medium between the two.

SK: Moving on again, is there a therapy we haven't mentioned that you feel is the most promising?

RM: Well no, but I'm very interested in all the energetic treatments that don't involve standard high-dose X-rays. There's great potential in using heat and light, microwaves, and other parts of the energy spectrum that are not as damaging as ionising radiation.

Hypothermia is something I've been interested in for a long time—fever therapy. But the actual practitioners of this therapy come and go, and you have to analyse everyone on a case-by-case basis. Photodynamic therapy is very promising.

These are the kind of therapies I would like to see expanded. Ionising radiation has such severe long-term and short-term side effects that it's more attractive to use low-dose radiation, or certain very targeted kinds of radiation. I think energy medicine in different forms is going to be the big thing in the future.

SK: Psychologically, what would you say to someone with cancer? I'm thinking here of someone, not with say stage one breast cancer, but someone much further down the line. What psychological message do you give to such people?

RM: I find the people who have a so-called philosophical attitude towards life do best. No one wants to die, no matter how old you are—people cling to life. But on the other hand, we all know that we all do die. So people who have incorporated that philosophical perspective and come to terms with it, and, whether they are religious or not, have some sort of spiritual outlook.

SK: Do you feel that such an attitude makes a place for healing?

RM: I do, because I think that if you're in a panic you're not going to heal. The fear factor can be so tremendous.

SK: I presume a lot of people come to you in a state of fear?

RM: We get individuals along the whole spectrum. Yesterday I spoke with somebody who was enormously calm in the face of everything. It's possible.

Sometimes when you're facing your greatest danger you become the calmest. For pleasure, at the moment I am reading Churchill's memoirs of World War Two. There is a very moving passage where he says that when war finally broke out, and he was given the admiralty position, that he suddenly felt this almost supernatural calmness. Before everything had become unbearably tense and dangerous but then there was this sort of incredible calm and peace. A kind of detachment from events that came over him and that really enabled him to do what he had to do.

He was the man who was more or less directing the whole of World War Two and probably had more pressure on him than any person on Earth. Yet the only way that he could deal with that was to reach this almost supernatural stage of acceptance. And because he experienced that, he was able to deal with these unbelievably frightening things.

He already knew about the pretension to nuclear bombs at this point—so he had that to worry about. When you think of the war and the potentials for worries that Churchill had…

SK: It's kind of—once you're in that calm then you can deal with things one step at a time.

RM: Exactly. And you can accept an innermost [feeling], no matter what may happen that there's also this sort of inner 'thy will be done' kind of mood. I think that when my clients have reached that point, that it is wonderful to work with them, because, in a detached way, we can stand back and say, 'well, let's look at this'.

SK: So you feel that overcoming fear is one of the most important factors?

RM: Oh I do, because if you're dealing out of fear and in a panic, I don't know how you can make good decisions.

I've seen the opposite, I've seen people absolutely stampeded and panicked by their disease. I don't blame them, but I think one has to pass through that and get to a place of being able to stand above it and see the whole picture.

It's hard, especially when you're dealing with people who have young children or where the cancer affects young children themselves. But para-doxically, the more you can stand outside and refuse to worry, the better decisions you can make.

SK: Well Ralph—this seems an appropriate place to end this interview as over-coming fear is open to absolutely everybody. Thank you very much for sharing your time and expertise.

RM: Thank you too.

7

Important Perspectives On Chemotherapy

O UR AIM IS TO ENCOURAGE you to utilise the most valuable approaches from both the conventional and unconventional worlds of cancer therapy. We urge you to straddle the divide that exists between the two, and to work past the antagonisms and rhetoric each side hurl at the other. We recommend you use your energies to discern the real efficacy of the various therapies on offer from both sides, and encourage you to consider the potential positives and negatives of each therapy you come across.

The cancer treatment field is full of contradictions, and what one professional states as certain and valuable is liable to be dismissed by another as unreliable and worthless. The fact is, that apart from certain cancers where proof of treatment has been proved beyond doubt, any course of action you take, conventional or unconventional, is likely to involve considerable risk. Cancer, for practitioners of both camps, is often a difficult disease to cure.

However, we do feel that Ralph Moss's advice, quoted earlier in the book is very important. Moss's states that he feels: 'it's important not to miss an opportunity just because of a revulsion to the bad side effects of a treatment. You want to make sure that where there is proof of an effectiveness of conventional treatment, that the person isn't over reacting and going headlong in the opposite direction'. An independent assessment of your chances with conventional treatment will help you make an informed decision, and we would again like to suggest that you obtain a Moss report on your particular cancer. (See p.5 for details.)

In recent decades, the end result (on the conventional side) of cancer proving such a 'difficult nut to crack' has been the ever-increasing use of highly toxic therapies. In part we can view this as representative of the sincere desire of health professionals wanting to do 'something' for individuals in their care—even when the odds of success are very low. 'Better offer something than nothing', or, 'better play safe and use a higher dosage', or, 'let's use everything we have at our disposal to fight the illness—even though the odds of success are low'. These are worthy and respectable sentiments and we must not forget that health professionals are faced with the task of dealing with thousands of individuals dealing with severe cases of cancer.

That said, over the last decade a clearer picture has been emerging about the end results of using highly toxic cancer treatments. The picture is not a pretty one—but even so, it is important we examine it well, so as to ensure you are able to make the most appropriate decisions. Specifically, the picture we need to examine is the use of high dose chemotherapy and/or extremely toxic procedures such as bone marrow transplants. From the beginning we will acknowledge that for some people these toxic treatments do yield results. However our concern in this section, surprisingly, is not with the successes obtained with these treatments, but with the rate of failure compared with success.

For instance, how many failures are there, what happens to an individual's quality of life when receiving a toxic treatment, and what damage is sustained to important organs of the body—in short, what is the overall cost paid by the unfortunate 'chemotherapy failures' for fortunate 'chemotherapy successes'? Specifically in this regard, our aim is to provide you with preliminary information, so that you can ascertain more clearly whether you actually stand to benefit from chemotherapeutic treatment, and how you can improve the chances of a successful outcome.

Anne E. Frahm, co-author of the self-help book, 'A Cancer Battle Plan', underwent surgery, followed by radiation, several gruelling regimes of chemotherapy, and finally a bone marrow transplant—all of which turned out to be in vain because her cancer kept returning. Anne describes the bone marrow transplant procedure in particular, as an experience nothing less than a living hell. In one particularly poignant passage she describes the physical and psychological state the bone marrow transplant left her in:

'The coughing and vomiting, which had become a major part of my hourly existence during these weeks and months, had caused my eyes to go bloodshot. My left eye was so completely red that no white was visible. It was real sci-fi! It didn't hurt much, but visitors would cringe when they first saw me. I'd also developed a rash that covered me from head to toe with deep reds and brilliant purples. My skin had been burned from the inside out, turning it eventually to a leathery brown. The outside layer of my mouth and gastrointestinal tract blistered and fell off. What a sight I must have been! Tubes running in and out of my "bald headed, bloody eyed, covered with splotches, decaying body." Yuck! Besides all these outer manifestations, the massive amounts of chemotherapy administered had taken a considerable toll internally. Damage was sustained to all my vital organs.'[50]

Worse was yet to come. When the results came back from the laboratory they indicated that the cancer still remained in Anne's body. After spending considerable time in the hospital trying her best to recover from the ordeal she had been through, Anne reports that she was in effect discharged and sent home to die, as nothing more could be done for her medically … Soon after, she began using the alternative approaches that she describes in her book. (The approaches Anne Frähm used are broadly similar to our Group 1 Therapies).

We are sure you also agree that treatment of the severity Anne Frähm received should not be entered into lightly. High dose chemotherapy regimes and bone marrow transplant procedures are extreme and intense treatments that can shatter the subtle and complex systems of the body. In case you're not familiar with a bone marrow transplant, let us run through a description of a typical treatment. First, stem cells are collected from the person who is to receive the therapy—they will be used later to 're-grow' their immune system. Stem cells are used in this regard because they have the ability to transform themselves into other more specialised cells needed for repair and maintenance of the body—specifically in this case, immune cells. The next stage of the therapy is the brutal part—high dosages of chemotherapy and radiation are directed at the tumour as well as at the individual's whole body. The aim is to kill off all rogue cancer cells that exist. However, this is no 'outpatient chemotherapy' where you might be able to function almost normally—this is as serious as it gets.

The therapy often continues until the patient's mind and body can take no more. For most individuals, this is a one-time therapy, so doctors tend to push as hard as they can to kill every last cancer cell. The problem, however, is that the treatment is not particularly cancer cell specific, and healthy cells end up being targeted and killed as well. The treatment targets cells that are dividing, because cancer cells (and all cells) are at their most vulnerable when they are transforming themselves from one cell into two cells. This is because the process of cellular division is an incredibly complex and delicate operation—for instance, the two metre long strand of DNA with its trillions of 'bits' of information, has to be split down the middle (one half for each cell) and then re-built up into a whole, in each of the two new cells.

If the rate of cancer cell division is much quicker compared with other cells, so much the better, because they will be more vulnerable, more often, compared with normal healthy cells. But with most cancers, the rate of cell division is similar to that of many other healthy cells in the body, and this makes healthy cells equally vulnerable to attack from the treatment. This is why the faster dividing cells of the mouth, throat lining, hair follicles and immune system are so often damaged even when there are no cancer cells in their immediate vicinity. This observation also ties in with the fact that the few cancers that respond well to chemotherapy are ones where the cancer cells do actually divide far more often than healthy cells.

A person receiving a bone marrow transplant needs to be kept completely isolated, because their immune system no longer functions and they are likely to pick up serious infections. The therapy continues for many days and causes much sickness—and people who have undergone the procedure report that all they can remember is just drifting in and out of consciousness, not really sure whether they are alive or dead.

Eventually, the chemotherapy and radiation treatments finish and the next phase of treatment begins. The previously collected stem cells are re-implanted back into the body with the hope they will quickly take hold and rebuild the individual's immune system. A while later, a test is performed to check if the procedure has been a success or a failure. If you remember the description of Anne Frähm's bone marrow transplant above—this was when the lab results came back indicating cancer cells were still present in her body.

To help you decide whether chemotherapy and/or extreme treatments are for you, the strategy we have chosen is to explain some of the concepts commonly used by medical professionals as well as some of the criticisms that have been made of chemotherapy in recent years by researchers such as Ralph Moss. It is hoped these explanations will enable you to make more sense of the information handed out by doctors and oncologists—or at least, that it will give you the confidence to check out exactly what they mean when they use 'medical phraseology'. We will also look at EVA® (Ex Vivo Apoptotic) testing, a procedure that can contribute to a better outcome of chemotherapy. The topics and the order we will cover them in are as follows:

1   EVA®

2   Surrogate measurements (Response rate, five-year survival, etc)

3   Survival rates and the impact of improved diagnosis

4   Other important criticisms of chemotherapy

EVA® (Ex Vivo Apoptotic Chemosensitivity Test): EVA® is not so much a critique of chemotherapy, but rather a method of dramatically improving the chances of a positive outcome. Unfortunately, at the present time, it is seldom used—the reason being that cancer professionals generally believe it is of no particular use. This kind of attitude is quite common, not necessarily because of arrogance on behalf of medical professionals, but because more often than not they are only familiar with the 'first generation' of a therapy or tool.

'First generations' of a therapy or 'tool' are often a prototype—a first go at something. However, it isn't long before a second or third generation version becomes available. We can see this happening at the present time in relation to photodynamic therapy—for instance if you asked an oncologist about photo-dynamic therapy or you looke it up on a cancer information database such as www.cancerbacup.org.uk, then most likely what you would read or hear about would be first generation photodynamic treatments and not later generation treatments such as the Cellular Light Therapy we have covered (see p.146). The same tends to happen with EVA®—the first generation tests suffered from obvious flaws, but there are now later generation, more accurate and more useful versions available.

Looking at the name, 'Ex Vivo Apoptotic', you may remember from a discussion earlier in the book about apoptosis, that it refers to a cell's timely death. 'Ex Vivo' refers to the fact that tumour cells from an individual's body are used for the tests (taken at time of biopsy or surgery), but are tested outside of the body in a laboratory environment. Specifically, the EVA® test examines which chemotherapy agents, and/or combinations of them, are most effective against a person's particular 'brand' of cancer cell. The test does this by measuring both the 'drug sensitivity' and the 'drug resistance' cells exhibit when exposed to a range of chemotherapeutic drugs. The data is then analysed to establish the chemotherapy regime most likely to work for the individual.

Knowing this information is invaluable, because it can save all the heartache of finding (or not finding) the same information through trial and error. Because chemotherapeutic agents are generally very toxic, and have such unpleasant side effects, they are not something any of us should take unless we

Problem	Solution
No Meaningful Increase in Patient Survival In The Last 45 Years	The EVA® assay measures drug induced cell death. Cell death measurements have correlated with patient response, time to progression and survival. By selecting the most effective treatments for individual patients, outcomes can be improved.
Patients receiving standardized 'cookie-cutter' therapies	EVA® assay-directed therapy diminishes the use of standardized regimens providing patient specific response profiles.
Toxic chemotherapy choices	EVA® assay-directed therapy reduces the use of ineffective drugs. If the right therapies are identified, potentially toxic, ineffective therapies can be avoided.
Slow, Costly, and Inefficient Drug Development	Drug development can be streamlined by using the EVA® assay to quickly identify the activity of new compounds in human cancer tissue. The EVA® assay targets drugs for the most responsive diseases.
Limited resources	The EVA® assay provides a cost-effective alternative to generic treatment programs by targeting resources toward the most effective chemotherapy treatment for each patient. The EVA® assay avoids therapeutic misadventures, diminishing futile care.

Table 11: EVA® Benefits[51]

are sure we are taking the right ones, and in the right combination. EVA® can help in this regard. Here is a table summarising its benefits for individuals dealing with cancer, as well as for oncologists and chemotherapists.

One issue raised about the results of the EVA® test is the following: 'Will drugs which are indicated as being more aggressive against a person's cancer be, ironically, more aggressive and toxic to that individual's body?' The answer we have been provided with is: 'We cannot control the toxicities of the chemotherapies. These are widely studied and well published. However, our goal is to determine which of many chemotherapeutics commit the tumour cells to apoptosis, or programmed cell death. From the list of agents that the patient's cancer cells are sensitive [to], the physician can then choose the ones that are the least toxic. Our goal, is [that] the most effective, least toxic regimen [is chosen] whenever chemotherapy is being recommended.'[52]

You can read detailed information about the EVA® test, including details about the tumour specimen required, as well as answers to other common

Type of cancer	Responses in %	Disease free survival in %
Breast stages III–IV	75	Rare
Small cell Lung Cancer	90	10
Stomach	50	Rare
Ovarian	75	10–20
Multiple Myeloma	75	Rare
Acute nonlymphatic leukemia	75	20
Chronic lymphocytic leukemia	75	Rare
Prostate	75	Rare
Head and Neck	75	Rare
Mycosis fungoides	75	Rare
Bladder	60	Rare

Table 12: % Response to Conventional Treatment vs. % Disease-Free Survival[53,54]

questions at www.rationaltherapeutics.com. The current cost of EVA® is £1562 ($2500).

SURROGATE MEASUREMENTS (RESPONSE RATE, DISEASE FREE SURVIVAL & FIVE-YEAR SURVIVAL RATE): Cancer professionals use their own particular terminology, and it is important you know what it means. For instance if an oncologist says to you, 'this chemotherapeutic agent has been shown to have an 80% response rate' then what exactly do they mean? Do they mean it has an 80% chance of curing the cancer, or of halting its progress, or some other meaning?

Actually, 'response rate' is a 'surrogate measurement' (substitute measurement) and generally refers to tumour shrinkage of 50% or more. This sounds like a very important measurement—but things are not quite as straightforward as they appear. As Ralph Moss has brought to light in 'Questioning Chemotherapy', response rate does not generally correlate with more important measurements such as increased life expectancy or disease free survival (i.e. length of time after treatment during which no cancer is found). The following tables illustrate the problem.

Type of Cancer	Statistics (White People)	Statistics (Black People)
Thyroid	94.7	90.2
Testis	93.6	87.3
Melanoma of the skin	85.3	70.3
Uterus	84.9	55.2
Breast (females)	81.6	65.8
Prostate gland	81.3	66.4
Urinary Bladder	80.7	30.0
Hodgkin's	79.4	74.1
Cervix Uterus	69.9	56.4
Larynx	69.1	53.1
Colon	60.9	49.7
Rectum	58.4	48.7
Kidney & Renal	56.9	52.0
Oral Cavity & Pharynx	54.6	33.6
Non-Hodgkin's	52.6	45.4
Ovarian	41.6	38.4
Leukaemia	39.5	30.8
Multiple Myeloma	27.4	29.4
Brain & Nervous System	26.7	30.6
Stomach	17.5	18.8
Lung & Bronchus	13.7	11.1
Oesophagus	10.5	6.1
Liver	6.6	4.0
Pancreas	3.0	4.9

Table 13: Five-Year Survival Rates in % (Source: National Cancer Institute)

As you can see, though the response rate (i.e. tumour shrinkage > 50%) to treatment can be high—even as high as 90% for small cell lung cancer—this does not correlate with a high chance of a period of disease free survival—only 10% for small cell lung cancer. A similar lack of correlation of response rate can occur for some cancers with another surrogate measurement—the five-year survival rate.

Putting the above tables together we can see, for instance, that ovarian cancer shows a 'response rate' of around 75%, a 10% – 20% chance of 'disease free survival', but a 'five-year survival' rate of between 38.4% and 41.6%. Prostate cancer, however, shows a 75% 'response rate', virtually no chance of a period of 'disease free survival', but a 66.4%–81.3% chance of 'five-year survival'. The point, therefore, we are trying to communicate is that these measurements (surrogate measurements) are able to disguise some of the hard reality of therapeutic outcome, in that each surrogate measurement by itself only represents one face or one aspect of the truth—and can therefore be misleading. A single surrogate measurement quoted on its own can be like a marketing or advertising man's best friend, in that even when the outlook is grim a high percentage figure can still be quoted to make everything seem 'rosier' than it really is.

The question we are most interested in is, how long do people live after they have received a certain treatment, and what quality of life do they experience? If we had clear answers to this question it would make comparing different therapies far simpler and more meaningful. However, for various reasons, oncologists have chosen to use substitute surrogate measurements (i.e. response rate, five-year survival and disease free survival, etc) rather than the length and quality of a person's life after therapy—and it is therefore important to appreciate surrogate measurements can be misleading if used inappropriately.

For instance, taking prostate cancer—from the figures above, we can't actually ascertain a person's quality of life. We can see that prostate cancer has a high response rate, and quite a high five-year survival rate, but except in rare instances the disease is nearly always going to remain, and therefore a person is likely to remain under treatment—with its possible side effects. Ongoing treatment raises questions about quality of life? Again, in the previous example of ovarian cancer—if a woman is told a likely response to chemotherapy will be 75%, it might sound so good that they may unhesitatingly sign up to a harsh and brutal therapeutic regime—when in fact their likely five-year survival rate is only around 40%.

Critics often point out that for medications that work consistently such as aspirin or antibiotics, surrogate measurements are rarely used. The implicit suggestion of this is that it is only when evidence of therapeutic success is thin on the ground that surrogate measurements begin to be utilised. Of course defenders of surrogate measurements claim there *is* a correlation between surrogate measurements and the all-important factor of length and quality of life lived—moreover that surrogate measurements make it easier to compare and quantify various therapies and treatments.

Our position is, there is truth to both sides, and that if a professional quotes a single surrogate type measurement to you, then you need to fill in the gaps and make sure you get a full picture of the situation. This is one reason we have recommended you obtain a report from Ralph Moss—as for any particular cancer, a more balanced and rounded appraisal of relevant statistics will be provided.

SURVIVAL RATES AND THE IMPACT OF IMPROVED DIAGNOSIS: Another important criticism of cancer statistics is the impact of improved diagnostics and screening for cancer upon the actual statistical survival rates.

Individuals often base their decision about receiving a conventional therapy upon statistical information they are given. However, it is important to understand that though the figures often sound attractive, they can mislead if they are not interpreted in the right way. Furthermore, 'raw statistics' can over look the impact of toxic side effects upon an individuals quality of life.

Let us look at the following scenario: twenty years ago, for a tumour to be detected during routine screening, it needed to be significantly more advanced (i.e. larger and more active). For example, it is estimated that breast cancer can now be detected around three years earlier than twenty years ago. Let's say, twenty years ago, a woman lived five years after diagnosis. Today, because of improved diagnosis (e.g. three years earlier for breast cancer), let us speculate that after diagnosis a woman lives eight years. From a superficial viewpoint, it appears survival rates have increased (from five years to eight years)—but as you can appreciate, this is not the case at all, rather this impression is given because the diagnosis has been made three years earlier.

This effect of improved diagnosis is known as 'lead-time bias'. It is obviously important to distinguish between a real improvement in therapeutic outcome and a superficial improvement in outcome figures, which can be explained by the 'lead-time bias' effect.

There is another phenomenon *caused* by the 'lead-time bias' effect. The effect is what Professor Alan Feinstein, one of the pioneers of cancer statistic analysis, has called stage migration. Feinstein noticed that the six-month survival rate of individuals dealing with lung cancer had jumped from 44% to 55% between the years of 1964 and 1977—despite there not being any significant advancement in treatment. His analysis of the survival rate identified that 'lead-time bias' was causing another knock-on effect.

Stage	Description
Stage I	Tumour is localised (often curable).
Stage II	Some spreading to nearby tissues or organs, but has not reached lymph nodes.
Stage III	Cancer has spread to local lymph nodes, but has not spread to distant parts of the body
Stage IV	Cancer has spread through the lymph system to distant organs and tissues of the body (often metastatic and inoperable).

*Note: There is also a more sophisticated staging system known as the TNM system. Staging systems in practice are quite specific for each kind of cancer.

Table 14: Universal Staging System*

You may be aware that a staging system is used to grade the severity of cancer. The stages commonly used (overall stage groupings) are as follows:

Feinstein identified that because of increased diagnostic tools, 'silent', non-active metastatic cancer was being identified earlier—yet because it was metastatic, it was being assigned to higher categories (III, or IV).

The effects of assigning individuals with 'non-active' metastatic cancer to higher categories means those individuals in categories III and IV, statistically now live longer (i.e. previously categories III and IV only contained individuals with 'active' metastatic cancer whereas now they contain individuals with 'non-active' metastatic cancer). Individuals in the lower categories (I & II) also live longer because these categories no longer contain individuals with non-active metastatic cancer (i.e. they only contain individuals with non-metastatic cancer).

This is a little complex to follow, and it is not essential that you understand it. What is essential, however, is that you are aware of the controversy surrounding the statistical claims made about chemotherapy treatments.

OTHER IMPORTANT CRITICISMS OF CHEMOTHERAPY: A few other important criticisms of chemotherapy are as follows:

Very few proper trials have ever been carried out comparing patients on chemotherapy with patients not on chemotherapy. Most studies only compare patients on one chemotherapy regime historically with patients on a different chemotherapy regime. The important point to note about comparative regime trials is that an underlying assumption is being made that chemotherapy is indeed effective i.e. that there is no need to compare individuals receiving chemotherapy with individuals not receiving any therapy whatsoever.

In the last seventy years chemotherapeutic treatment has shown definite and indisputable increases in survival time with only a few types of cancer. These cancers are, 'acute lymphatic leukaemia, Hodgkin's disease, testicular and ovarian cancer, and a handful of rare tumours, mainly of childhood'.[55] Many others cancers appear as though they have improved survival rates in comparison with previous years, but further examination of the data often indicates that this is due to lead-time bias—as discussed above.

Individuals who have undergone treatment report chemotherapy can be a terrible and frightening experience. It violates the Hippocratic oath regarding the principle of doing no harm. Often extensive damage occurs to organs such as the bone marrow and the liver during treatment. The toxicity of chemotherapy destroys the body's natural immune system when a patient needs it most, thereby making them more susceptible to secondary cancer. The whole approach of chemotherapy is totally opposite to that of employing a non-toxic (non-harming) approach and supporting the body to heal itself.

Large numbers of people are enrolled into chemotherapy treatment when in fact there is no real evidence that it helps their condition. For instance, an analysis of the figures indicate that nine out of ten women who only receive surgery for early stage breast cancer will not have a recurrence within five years (the standard yardstick to be considered a cure)—yet almost a 100% of the women diagnosed with early stage breast cancer will be recommended to follow a course in chemotherapy—even though a reading of the above figures show that only 10% of women might benefit (i.e. for the above example—100% of women taking chemotherapy when it is likely to only help 10% of them).[56]

Trial phase	Description
Phase I	Designed to test the safety of a particular drug in human beings. Might include an attempt at identifying the optimum dose and route of administration.
Phase II	Designed to find out more about the safety of a new treatment and to examine the efficacy of the treatment against one or a number of cancer types.
Phase III	This phase involves more individuals than earlier phases and compares one group receiving the new treatment with another group receiving a placebo.

Table 15: Different phases of clinical trials

With regard to enrolling on a clinical trial (something that is offered to large numbers of people), our view is that it may sound flattering or altruistic, but in terms of quality of life it might not be in your interest to participate. Below is a list of the different trial phases that commonly take place:

If you enrolled in a phase 1 trial, it would mean you would be acting as a guinea pig in terms of establishing an optimal dose of a new drug (i.e. no one really knows how bad the side effects could be of a particular dose, never mind whether it will provide any direct therapeutic benefit for you). A phase 3 trial might be a better bet as optimum and safe dosages have already been ascertained in the previous phases—however, in a well run trial you wouldn't necessarily know which arm of the study you would be enrolled on, whether on the arm receiving the new treatment or the arm receiving an older treatment or one receiving no treatment at all. Of course there is the chance that enrolling on a particular trial could work out well for an individual—but again it is important that you are aware of the issues surrounding enrolment. In terms of research and the drug companies, you are a valuable commodity. As people are becoming more informed about the possible downside of enrolling in a trial, it is becoming harder and harder for the big multinationals to recruit suitable candidates.

Action of chemotherapy

As we approach the end of this section it is worth considering the way in which chemotherapy is used, and for what reasons. As has been mentioned in previous sections of the book, the main problem with cancer is that it metastasises (spreads) around the body. At any one time, it is estimated that there are millions of rogue cancer cells floating around in the blood stream of an individual with active malignant cancer. These can settle down in a particular area of the body and start growing—though as John Boik pointed out, for this to happen requires a cell to pass through a set of remarkably complex steps (see p.34). Chemotherapy is often used as an attempt to kill all of the rogue cells—the theory being that if all the cancer cells are killed the cancer will come to an end. However, the problem chemotherapists face is that it only requires one cell to start the whole cancer problem off again.

The harsh reality is it is very difficult to kill every last cancer cell in the body, especially without damaging an individual's immune system. We should remember that ideally, the best agent to kill every last cancer cell is an individual's own immune system—this is the job it has carried out successfully for all the years before cancer developed. That is why so many non-toxic therapies veer towards supporting and enhancing the immune system and it is the greatest irony of chemotherapy that it can leave an individual's immune system completely shattered.

Of course, in the end, maybe you will decide to receive chemotherapy—even though the odds are not stacked in your favour. It is difficult to say no when it is recommended by the professionals we have been brought up to respect and consider knowledgeable. However, if you do decide to receive chemotherapy, there is no reason why you cannot combine it with other non-toxic immune supporting therapies (such as those we have discussed in this book). There are many indications that the overall therapeutic effect of chemotherapy is enhanced when the two approaches are combined. (It is worth noting that the same applies to all three of the main conventional approaches—surgery, radio-therapy and chemotherapy. Surgery, if the cancer is operable, is generally considered to be the most effective of the conventional approaches, especially if the cancer is detected at an early stage). Certainly many chemotherapy depart-ments now routinely suggest individuals supplement their diet with antioxi-dants—something they would have scoffed at several years ago. Moss presents a simple list of antioxidants considered suitable for individuals to take during chemotherapy treatment. They are as follows:

Antioxidant	Preventative Dose	Therapeutic Dose
Beta-carotene	15mg	45mg
Bioflavonoids	2 grams	8 grams
Coenzyme Q10	100mg	400mg
Glutathione*	250mg	1000mg
N-Acetyl Cysteine*	600mg	2400mg
Non beta-carotine carotenoids (e.g. lycopene)	15mg	45mg
Selenium	250 µg	750 µg
Vitamin C	2 grams	10 grams
Vitamin E	400 IU	1600 IU

* There are better methods of raising glutathione levels—see discussion on p.21 for details.

Table 16: Leibovitz's Antioxidant Formula[57]

It is also worth pointing out that John Boik discusses 'Natural Compounds, Chemotherapy, and Radiotherapy' in detail in his book if you would like more information.[58]

Lastly in this section we would like to reiterate that a personalised report (see p.5) and second opinions are vital in terms of obtaining the necessary information to make the best decision about chemotherapy. Please obtain as much information as possible about your chances with the choices available—and from independent sources. Always remember that toxic treatments may reduce your options in the future because of the damage they can cause your immune system.

8

Beginning & Continuing

WE ARE NOW APPROACHING the end of the main part of our study (though you will find some more interesting and useful material in appendices A, B & C). We have looked at a number of different therapies that are available, and it is hoped you have already started, or are preparing to start, several of them. We hope you will use a 'spread' of therapies from all of the three groups, and that you will definitely employ at least one of the Group 3 Therapies. Also, regardless of any other actions you take, we hope you will seek out second opinions, as well as invest in a report from Ralph Moss. Then, you will have the best available information from which to work with.

We should not forget that individuals who utilise conventional, unconventional or a mix of therapies, and who go on to overcome cancer are often very committed and prepared to put in significant effort. That said, there is no reason why, overall, this cannot be an interesting and exhilarating experience. Of course, at times you may feel down, unmotivated and sceptical that anything positive can be achieved. This is only natural, but as medical herbalist Dr. Richard Schulze clearly emphasises, you should never give up. Whatever the outlook, keep struggling and stay determined to win through. In this vein, what has surprised us most while we have been writing this book, are the many reports of elderly people recovering from secondary cancers. It is generally easier to ascribe the powers of healing to young people rather than to older people—but in fact there are many reliable accounts of very elderly people overcoming cancer (or living with it) and living for many years beyond what was expected at the time of diagnosis.[59]

Cancer is an illness which often demands dedication, and a significant change in lifestyle, if it is to be overcome or 'coaxed back into the fold' (see p.34). A few herbal teas and an occasional session of a relevant therapy aren't likely to be enough. So, though at this stage it might seem overwhelming, in many senses, there is no reason why you should not aim to build a significant number of the therapies we have discussed into your lifestyle. Usually cancer takes many years to germinate, and during this time many factors build up in the body that allow cancer to continue forming. The fact is that when cancer has formed, several systems of the body have not been able to properly carry out their correct function—or the environment of the body has not been conducive to efficient working of the body's various protective systems. In this regard, cancer should be seen as a systemic disease (i.e. a whole body illness). Though it may break out in the 'weakest' and most vulnerable location, it should be viewed that an individual's whole body is in need of a good service and overhaul. This service or overhaul should address all areas of life: eating, sleeping, supplemental nutrients, mind-body connection and all the other areas addressed by the therapies we have discussed. For recovery from cancer—it is best to use a fully comprehensive approach, addressing the illness on many different fronts. Moreover, to be life-changing the therapy should be intensive. (It is worth bearing in mind that 'nature' often employs approaches with built-in redundancy—that is, if one particular strategy to defeat illness should only half work, then another fallback strategy is immediately available to complete the task). However, in contrast to what we have just said, we also want to stress that we feel it is important that you do not become fanatical about your therapies and lifestyle. We feel it is important that you maintain some sort of balance between the efforts you put into healing and other areas of your life.

Utilising the majority of therapies we have discussed is going to be quite costly. However it is likely that some individuals will manage to carry out many of the therapies we have covered even though they have very little money or resources. We therefore have to take the position that if the determination is present, then a way will be found to achieve it. Cancer is both a frightening and a fascinating subject—and every single person around you has a direct interest in seeing you succeed. It is probably only a matter of time before one of their loved ones succumbs to the illness. Why not build on this and ask for help and support from those around you. And most importantly—feel that you deserve the best, and are worth it. Of course, at the same time, you should recognise that making lifestyle changes can be a challenging task—and therefore you should not scold yourself too harshly if sometimes it all feels a bit too much.

We should acknowledge that we have presented alternative and unconventional therapies in a positive and optimistic light, indicating that they can form an important part of your anti-cancer program either on their own or in conjunction with conventional therapies. Sooner or later, however, you are likely to come across other less generous perspectives. Such viewpoints might come from a medical professional, or you might read them in a magazine or on a website.

You should note that existing conventional cancer treatments are estimated to be worth around two hundred billion dollars per year[60]—and because of this you should not underestimate the lengths to which existing business interests are prepared to go to protect their income stream. Additionally, though it is slowly changing, in the past, cancer institutions have shown themselves to be deeply hostile and suspicious towards unconventional therapies.

In 1991, for example, supported by a large grant from the National Cancer Institute (NCI), retired researcher Saul Green, published a series of articles on unconventional cancer therapies. The justification for the articles was that they would serve as a useful 'educational' resource for individuals seeking to find out more about unconventional treatments. In the articles Green, by presenting 'facts' 'selectively', 'articulately' though often incorrectly, wrote in a totally damning way about many unconventional therapies. Not content with consigning unconventional therapies to the rubbish bin, Green bolstered his position by personally attacking and mocking the discoverers and founders of many alternative therapies, attempting to make them seem like charlatans, frauds and quacks.

Of course there are charlatans 'out there', but Green's targets were scientists and researchers who had dedicated their lives (and life-savings) to solving the riddle of cancer—not fast talking conmen trying to make a fast buck. It is difficult here, to summarise the intensity and bitterness of the battle that has raged between the conventional and unconventional camps—and how unfair and arrogant the establishment's attitude has been over recent decades. If you are interested in reading more about this subject, please see Ralph Moss's The Cancer Industry.

As Moss stated in the interview with him (see p.167), 'dogs bark but the caravan moves on'. Moss is of the opinion that quackbuster' like Saul Green or Stephen Barrett (of Quackwatch) have lost the war between conventional and unconventional therapies. In the end they have been proved wrong. Actually, because they were so extreme and one-sided in their viewpoints, it was only a matter of time before they 'lost'. Over recent decades, 'The Quackbusters' have even mocked therapies with thousands of years of experience such as acupuncture and Chinese herbal medicine—in fact any health therapy not accepted by conventional authorities. We can view their actions as part of a determined and ruthless campaign run in the 1980's and 90's to 'nip' unconventional therapies in the bud.

However, even though the therapies they attacked such as Burzynski's Antineoplastons or Burton's IAT therapy—have all shown themselves (in best case series or other studies) to exert anti-tumour effects the 'Quackbusters' propaganda lives on—and still misleads with its ferocity and selective presentation of facts. The Quackbusters were relying on individuals outside the research having little power or ability to determine whether an article written in a scientific or scholarly way is either true or false—and most likely, people will think it is true. So, if you do come across such writings, our advice is to consult with someone like Moss—someone who is trying to seriously determine the truth about the potency of each therapy—before you accept what the article describes. Also there are some good refutations of Green's articles on Antineoplastons and Burton's IAT therapy in 'The Burzynski Breakthrough' by Thomas D. Elias (General Publishing Group:1997) and 'Alternatives in Cancer' by Penelope Williams (Key Porter Books: 2000).

We decided to end the book with a couple of short anecdotes, which we feel convey some important truths. We have hesitated to include these, as we have worried they will trivialise all that we have covered. However, on reflection we feel they are unusual and have decided to include them after all. If anything, they belong to the category of 'mind and body' because they are stories which linger in the mind and exert a positive influence.

The first anecdote relates to a woman who was scheduled to have a mastectomy. Her surgery was running late and in an unusual set of circumstances she found herself parked on a trolley outside the operating theatre, not yet having received her full anaesthetic.

The women described how as she lay there, a nurse awkwardly and hurriedly burst out from the double doors of the operating theatre. Something about the air of the nurse caused the lady on the trolley to look more closely at what she was carrying in her hand.

As she looked more closely she saw that the nurse was carrying a clear plastic bag, smeared with blood, and that it contained a large bloody breast of a woman that looked as though it had been hacked off her body. This moment proved decisive, and the woman determined right there and then that there was no way that anyone was going to do that to her body. She promised herself as resolutely as possible that one way or another she would beat her illness—and got straight up off the trolley, cancelled the operation and went home. It is related that she did indeed find the appropriate resources she needed, and did later fully recover.

We can interpret this first anecdote to illustrate the power of pure determination and the will to heal—and to find different ways to achieve healing. The second anecdote, however, illustrates a different aspect of healing. This story relates to an Indian woman who came in for surgery regarding discomfort in her abdomen. The surgeon described that when he opened her up, he found that she was full of cancerous tissue. So much in fact, that he felt there was nothing he could do. He therefore stitched her back up and went to speak with the family to explain the bad news.

Her family had, of course, been very concerned about the operation, but after the surgeon told the family what he had found they pleaded with him not to tell the truth about the cancer to their mother. The surgeon reports that, much to the detriment of his supposed professional integrity, he did allow himself to be persuaded by the family and so later told his patient that he had found nothing serious during the operation and that she would be absolutely fine within a few weeks.

The surgeon had of course expected that she would die very soon after. However he found out much later that the woman was still living and was in fact very healthy. It was as though the profound relief she experienced at finding out that nothing was wrong with her created an environment conducive to healing.

Though admittedly unusual, 'miracles' like this do happen—there are many such documented and medically accepted cases referred to as 'spontaneous regressions'.[61]

All that remains for us now is to thank you for taking the time to read this information and to wish you well in your journey to find health. Please write to us with you experiences, questions and details of new cancer treatments and/or advances you come accross. You can reach us at: authors@healing-cancer.co.uk.

Please take time to read the appendices as well, especially:

- Appendix A: Additional Well Known Cancer Therapies
- Appendix B: Important Theories Of Cancer
- Appendix C: Useful Contacts & Resources

Most likely you will find the information just as valuable as the information in the main part of the book.

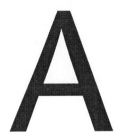

Appendix A: Additional Well Known Cancer Therapies

W E HAVE INCLUDED information about some other commonly used cancer therapies in this appendix—specifically popular herbal remedies for cancer and mega-vitamin C therapy. In the case of herbal remedies such as essiac, it is here in the appendix because we feel it has been superseded by the information presented in 'Natural Anti-Tumour Compounds Discussed By John Boik' (p.34). In the case of mega-vitamin C therapy, it is here because earlier in the book we recommended one to two grams per day as the optimum amount. However there are other schools of thought who consider much higher dosages are warranted.

Rene Caisse & Other Herbal Remedies

On first hearing it is easy to dismiss Rene Caisse's herbal 'tea' remedy for cancer as simply inadequate. Somehow, the idea of a 'tea' for cancer just doesn't seem appropriate for such a fearful adversary and potentially fatal illness.

However, over the years Rene Caisse's herbal decoction known as essiac (Caisse backwards) has been used by hundreds of thousands of individuals dealing with cancer, many of whom claim that it has been responsible for a significant improvement, or even cure, of their cancer. There are literally thousands of testimonials attesting to the value of essiac tea. For these reasons it is important to examine Rene Caisse's herbal remedy to see what it can offer us as a cancer therapy and as a cancer preventative.

Rene Caisse first heard about the tea early in her career while nursing a woman with particularly prominent scar tissue on one of her breasts. The lady explained to Rene that over thirty years earlier she had been diagnosed with advanced breast cancer and been offered a mastectomy by conventional doctors. However, an American Indian healer, whom the lady knew, suggested that instead of a mastectomy she should try an ancient Indian remedy. The lady decided to take the Indian remedy instead of a mastectomy, all went well and she fully recovered. Caisse writes:

> 'She was nearly eighty years old when I saw her and there had been no recurrence of cancer. I was much interested and wrote down the names of the herbs she had used. I knew that the doctors threw up their hands when cancer was discovered in a patient; it was the same as a death sentence, [or] just about. I decided that if I should ever develop cancer, I would use this herb tea.'[62]

After receiving the recipe from this elderly lady, another incident occurred to Rene about a year later. Caisse describes how she was taking a walk with a retired doctor when he reached down and showed her a common weed. Caisse writes:

> '[The doctor] told me, "If people would use this weed there would be very little cancer in the world." He told me the name of the plant. It was one of the herbs my patient named as an ingredient of the Indian medicine man's tea!'[63]

Rene's curiosity about the value of the herbal mix had been aroused. Beginning with her aunt and progressing case by case under the supervision of various doctors, Rene Caisse began treating cancer patients using the herbal formula. Before long, Rene had accumulated many successful case histories and demonstrated remarkable results.

Suitably impressed, the group of eight doctors supervising Rene's work, presented a petition to the Department of Health in Ottawa stating the following:

'Dated at Toronto on October 27, 1926:

To Whom It May Concern:

We the undersigned believe that the 'Treatment for Cancer' given by Nurse R.M. Caisse can do no harm and that it relieves pain, will reduce the enlargement and will prolong life in hopeless cases. To the best of our knowledge, she has not been given a case to treat until everything in medical and surgical science has been tried without effect and even then she was able to show remarkable beneficial results on those cases at that late stage.

We would be interested to see her given an opportunity to prove her work in a large way. To the best of our knowledge she has treated all cases free of any charge and has been carrying on this work over the period of the past two years.

(Signed by the eight doctors)'[64]

Soon after this petition was submitted, the authorities delivered their response: Caisse was arrested for practicing medicine without a licence—an event she describes as marking the beginning of fifty years of persecution by various authorities.

Rene Caisse's remedy can be viewed as representing a 'herbal' approach to cancer—one whose roots stretch back to traditional American Indian civilization, where it formed part of the natural wisdom of the culture. Further, Caisse herself constantly refined the remedy, in terms of its ingredients and the proportion of each used, until she was satisfied she had identified the optimum medicine to benefit her patients. It would seem that Caisse, though not a formally trained herbalist, had an intuitive grasp of the powerful yet subtle strength that nature can offer us in healing.

Of great significance is the fact that Rene Caisse treated some forty thousand individuals dealing with advanced and terminal cancer over a forty-year period. Caisse carried out this work virtually single-handedly and asked only for voluntary financial contributions from her patients. A nurse by training, Caisse undoubtedly deserves the greatest of praise for her determination, her perseverance and the many actual often-documented improvements her experienced. Rene Caisse was very much a devoted servant of the people in the same tradition as Florence Nightingale and Mother Teresa—combining humble service with immense practical experience to bring about improvement in the lives of suffering individuals. Caisse wrote the following concerning the benefits she considered essiac to possess:

> 'If it does not cure cancer it will afford relief, if the patient has suffi-cient vitality remaining to enable him to respond to treatment.'[65]

And after examining Rene Caisse's documentation of her work, including X-rays, Dr Banting, the discoverer of insulin, told her:

> 'Miss Caisse... I will not say you have a cure for cancer. But you have more evidence of a beneficial treatment for cancer than anyone in the world.'[66]

So what does Rene Caisse's remedy consist of, and how can you go about obtaining it? We should note from the outset that incorporating Caisse's herbal decoction as one of your complementary cancer therapies should only cost you in the region of £5 ($8) per month. However, many companies will attempt to extract far more from you– maybe even several hundred dollars a month. (We will list some low cost sources later).

The actual ingredients and their proportions in the recipe have been the subject of much interest and controversy. Caisse was an immensely secretive person and for over fifty-five years limited the knowledge of her formula to only a few trusted friends and colleagues. Caisse claims she kept the formula secret because she feared that the authorities would either systematically destroy its reputation or leave it on the shelf if she revealed its ingredients—just as she considered they had done with Pasteur's smallpox vaccine that took fifty years to be accepted. This was not purely paranoia on her behalf. Treating so many patients, and obtaining such unheard-of results gave Rene Caisse an unprece-dented reputation as a person capable of healing terminal and advanced cases of cancer—a reputation the medical authorities of the day were none too pleased about. This resulted in Caisse coming under immense pressure, with hearings on her remedy and legal right to treat cancer patients going right to the top of Canadian state institutions.

There has been a great deal of debate and speculation as to the exact formu-lation of Rene's essiac herbal decoction. As Sheila Snow and Mali Klein describe in their excellent book, *Essiac – The secrets of Rene Caisse's Herbal Pharmacy*, it appears that even when Caisse did occasionally divulge essiac's ingredients to others, she always altered them slightly from her own tried and tested formula. Therefore, after much research, Snow and Klein report the formula employed by Rene Caisse herself to consist of the following:[67]

- Powdered Sheep Sorrel (whole plant including roots and seeds)
- Burdock Root (chopped into small pieces—'pea' size)

- Powdered Slippery Elm inner bark
- Powdered Turkey Rhubarb root

The preparation process for these ingredients is as follows. Note that we will give instructions for fifty grams total of the four herb dried mix. This will make sufficient essiac for one person for just over two months. We have used fifty grams because the herbs are often offered in this or a similar 2oz measure quantity.[68]

1 The ingredients should be mixed thoroughly together.

2 Broken down, the mix is 26.6g Burdock Root, 17.7g Sheep Sorrel, 4.4g Slippery Elm inner bark and 1.1g Turkey Rhubarb root (corresponding ratios 24:16:4:1).

3 Take a large pot (stainless steel or enamel) and boil 1.6 litres of water (ratio of herb mix to water is 1:32).

4 Add herb mix and cover pot with tight fitting lid and boil hard for ten minutes.

5 Turn off the heat and make sure that any herbs left stuck on the side of the pot are pushed down from the side of the pot into the mixture.

6 Leave for twelve hours (preferably on a warm plate)—with the pot lid on.

7 Then heat until steaming hot but not boiling.

8 Turn off heat and strain liquid through a fine strainer into warm sterilised bottles.

9 Immediately seal and store in a dark cupboard.

How to take essiac

Using essiac is very simple. 30ml of essiac diluted in a cup of warm water should be drunk every night, on an empty stomach, before bed. The therapy can be carried on for many years, though it is suggested that after long term use it should only be taken three weeks out of every four so as to keep up the body's response to the herbs. Any open bottles of essiac should be stored in the fridge since there are no preservatives in the formula. Also Caisse considered it important not to increase the 30ml dose as this is the dose she found worked the best, the use of any more provided no additional benefit.

What about the Eight Herb Recipe?

You will often see references to an eight-herb essiac recipe. Ingredients commonly used to make up the additional four ingredients are:

- Cleavers
- Gold Thread
- Periwinkle
- Red Clover
- Watercress
- Blessed Thistle
- Kelp

In their investigations, however, Snow and Klein see no reason to include any of the above. It would seem that early in her career Caisse did include certain of the above herbs, but later discarded them as her research into an optimal formula continued. Furthermore, Red Clover is advised against for anyone with a hormonal based cancer—it is a herb containing oestrogen and might therefore stimulate an oestrogen dependant cancer. We therefore recommend you seek out the original four-herb formula mix of essiac.

The most important ingredient of essiac would seem to be Sheep Sorrel. This is the herb that Rene's research found to have the most profound anti-cancer action. Caisse included the other three herbs as 'support' for the Sheep Sorrel. She considered that as the Sheep Sorrel causes the tumour to regress, dead cells and other waste matter left over from the tumour circulate around the body and place it under increased stress. The other three herbs therefore act as blood purifiers and help with detoxification. In fact, Caisse obtained her best results when using a special purified (of protein) decoction of Sheep Sorrel, delivered to individuals via intramuscular injection around the site of their tumour. Caisse used intramuscular injections in conjunction with the oral four-herb medicine. However, you should *never* inject any decoction that you produce— as without proper and complete processing it could cause a severe reaction and even death.

It is often described that essiac can help draw secondary cancer cells back to the site of an original tumour. As you will recall, it is rare that an individual's primary tumour causes death, but rather death is usually caused by secondary tumours appearing in other parts of the body. The success of surgery is directly related to this point—if a tumour can be removed as a complete whole, and none of its microscopic 'spidery' tentacles left behind, then an individual will often have a good outlook. So if it is true that essiac does help draw cancer cells back to the original site, then it is indeed a very valuable therapy.

Does Rene Caisse's herbal remedy work?

This of course is the most important question. Certainly from animal experiments she conducted, Caisse demonstrated that her formula has a beneficial effect. She reports:

> '[I worked] on mice at the Christie Street Hospital Laboratories in Toronto, with Dr. Norich and Dr. Lockhead. I did so from 1928 through 1930. These mice were inoculated with Rous Sarcoma. I kept the mice alive fifty-two days, longer than anyone else had been able to do, and in later experiments with two other doctors, I kept mice alive for seventy-two days with essiac.'[69]

Several doctors visited Caisse's clinic to ascertain whether essiac worked. A Dr Richard Leonardo, a surgical specialist, was sceptical at first but after four days at the clinic examining patients and records he stated to Rene:

> 'Young lady … I must congratulate you. You have made a wonderful discovery. I like your method of treatment … I feel it will change the whole theory of cancer treatment and will eventually do away with surgery, radium and X-ray treatments for cancer.'[70]

Also a Dr Emma Carson visited the clinic and stayed a total of sixteen days. She writes about what she saw:

> 'When I arrived in Bracebridge, I contemplated remaining twelve hours, at least not more than forty-eight hours. Miss Caisse and her ESSIAC treatment and her patients were responsible for the unlimited extension of my time in Bracebridge and Toronto, as I remained twenty-four days and spent about sixteen days at Toronto.
>
> During the three weeks of the time I visited Bracebridge and neighbouring cities and towns, I examined and investigated results obtained by ESSIAC treatments including four hundred patients.

The vast majority of Miss Caisse's patients were brought for treatment after surgery, radium, X-rays, etc. had failed to be helpful and the patients pronounced incurable or hopeless cases. Really, the progress obtainable and the actual results from ESSIAC treatments and the rapidity of repair were absolutely marvellous, and must be seen to convincingly confirm belief.'[71]

The above reviews of Rene Caisse's work are undoubtedly very positive and upbeat. It should be borne in mind, however, that no properly run human trials have been carried out. It should also be borne in mind that from a psychological point of view, Caisse created an environment particularly conducive to healing. You will remember earlier that we mentioned that being a member of a therapeutic group can significantly impact on survival time. In another part of her statement, Dr Carson describes the 'atmosphere' of the clinic. She writes:

> 'I had never before seen or been in any manner associated with such a remarkably cheerful and sympathetic clinic, regardless of size, location or number of persons; or attended a more peaceful, sympathetic clinic anywhere.'[72]

John Boik (see p.34) is not so sure how useful remedies such as essiac are—from the point of view that they only contain very low amounts of active anti-cancer substances.[73] You will recall that Boik has identified a number of natural compounds that can exert a beneficial action with regard to cancer. He would agree that herbal cancer remedies such as essiac do indeed contain compounds beneficial in respect of cancer—but that these compounds are better taken in far larger amounts (and along with a greater number of complementary compounds to increase the magnification achieved through synergism). Certainly, from his calculations, there simply isn't anywhere near enough of any active ingredient in each dose of essiac to make a significant impact on cancer cells. (Note: Of course, there is the possibility the body responds to the 'quality' or 'essence' of a remedy rather than quantity—but this is still speculation and not yet proven).

As regards the compatibility of essiac with other therapies—certainly essiac is absolutely fine to use in conjunction with all the other therapies we have described, and also all mainstream cancer therapies. Snow and Klein themselves recommend essiac is best combined with other naturopathic health-building therapies (Group 1 Therapies).

The Harry Hoxsey Remedy

Another well-known formula is Harry Hoxsey's herbal remedy. Interestingly (as the remedy is thought to be another product of ancient American Indian culture) several of its ingredients have been found to possess anti-cancer action in laboratory studies. The full list of herbal ingredients for Hoxsey's internal tonic is as follows:

- Liquorice
- Red Clover

- Burdock Root

- Stillingnia Root

- Barberis Root

- Poke root

- Cascara Sagrada

- Prickly ash bark

Hoxey's tonic is available ready prepared in tonic form but for some reason, from only a few suppliers. You will find a supplier listed later in this section.

Herb Shield – Alan Hopkins

Other practitioners such as Alan Hopkins recommend a more comprehensive herbal approach. His Herb Shield contains the following:

In this concoction, certain of the herbs have been shown to have definitive anti-cancer action while others are supportive of the immune system in general and some are considered restorative herbs that rebalance and restore the body's normal function.

In terms of the 'manufacture' of the tonic, all the herbs are first individually prepared as tinctures. This means the herbs are soaked in a mixture of organic alcohol and water for at least one month (no heat is applied—so no constituents are lost). Each herb is then pressed and the Herb Shield Tonic is made from the fluid extracts using specific percentages of each herb.

Within the herbal field, some traditional practitioners oppose such a 'comprehensive' mixing of herbs—their main objection being that the herbs do not grow together in nature in a complementary way—instead coming from many different and disparate parts of the world. (Traditional herbalism views plants and herbs growing together in nature as mutually supportive of each other). Hopkins, however, is confident that his approach is taking the practice of herbalism into the 21st century. He considers the fact they do not grow together in nature as secondary to the scientific work that has been carried out in recent years examining the biological activity of differing herbs. Such an approach is certainly more in line with Boik's recommendations and because of its large number of ingredients, Herb Shield will benefit from the magnification effects of synergism.

It is worth noting a few facts about one of the Herb Shield's ingredients—Mistletoe. Mistletoe is used as a cancer therapy in its own right by therapists who follow the anthroposophical teachings of Rudolph Steiner. The Mistletoe is fermented into a preparation known as Iscador, which has been shown to stimulate the immune system and increase white blood cell counts.[73] It is remarkable Mistletoe was identified by 'herbalism' as an immune-stimulating compound many years before it was shown to have such properties in a laboratory. Steiner reputedly identified Mistletoe as anti-cancerous because the plant itself acts like a cancer on the tree upon which it grows; for instance Mistletoe grows in all directions, and without any order; it grows and flowers when it feels like it; and lastly, it acts like a parasite on the tree, sending its feeders into branches to suck out vital nutrients. A recommended clinic specialising in this therapy is the Humlegaarden Clinic in Denmark (www.humlegaarden.dk).

Cost:

Essiac: £5 ($8.00) / month
Hoxsey herbal type mix: £18.13 ($29) / month
Herb Shield: £23.95 ($38.32) / month

Herbal Ingredients of 'Herb Shield'		
Ashwagandha root	Garlic bulb	Psoralia seed
Astragalus root	Golden Thread root	Raspberry leaf
Barbat Skullcap herb	Korean Ginseng root	Red Clover flower
Bilberry fruit	Liquorice root	Rhubarb root
Black Walnut leaf / husks	May Apple root	Schizandra berry
Blood root	Milk Thistle root	Scutellaria barbata root
Cat's claw bark	Mistletoe leaf	Sheep Sorrel herb
Chapperal herb	Myrrh gum	Suma root
Cleavers herb	Nettle root	Sweet Violet leaf
Condurango bark	Oldenlandia stems	Tabebuia bark
Dandelion leaf	Olive Tree leaf	Thorn Apple leaf
Echinacea root	Periwinkle tops	Thuja leaf
Fresh wheatgrass & high chlorophyll herbs	Poke root	Tumeric root

Table 17: Alan Hopkins 'Herb Shield'

Where to obtain the formulas/herbs

Essiac: You will find a chart comparing the price of essiac from many suppliers around the world at: http://essiac-info.org/prices.html. It is recommended you find a supplier who uses organic grade herbs.

Metabolics in the UK do an essiac tincture to be taken 5–20 drops 3 times per day before meals mixed with a small amount of water. Costs £5.64 ($10.15) for 30ml.

Metabolics Ltd.
5 Eastcott Common
Eastcott
Devizes
Wiltshire
SN10 4PL

☎: +44 (0) 1380 812799
📠: +44 (0) 1380 813078
Email: sales@metabolics.co.uk

Hoxsey herbal mix: www.herbmed.com offer a product called Red Clover/Burdock Plus which contains the Hoxsey herbs and more. It is estimated that a 4 oz bottle (taking fifteen to forty-five drops, two to three times daily between meals) will last a month.

Metabolics in the UK offer a Hoxey tincture (20% alcohol) to be taken 5–20 drops 3 times per day before meals mixed with a small amount of water. See above for address. Costs £10.25($18.45) for 30ml.

Herb Shield: Alan Hopkins at www.godshaer.co.uk

Vitamin C in Cancer Therapy

Many doctors employing unconventional cancer approaches attest to the power of mega-vitamin C therapy. You are probably aware vitamin C is beneficial for teeth and gums, that it prevents scurvy and that it acts as a general antioxidant in the body. You have probably noticed it being included in food products as a preservative or as a nutrient enhancer—for example, in breakfast cereals it is used to replace some of the vitamin content processed out during the manufacturing process. What you are probably not aware of are some of the startling results obtained when using it in mega-dose levels as a therapy for cancer. In this section we will explore these issues—but first consider the following:

Are you aware that nearly all living beings—*except* humans, primates, monkeys, guinea pigs, the trout and a few other animals—all synthesise their own vitamin C in large quantities? For example, a goat weighing 70kgs synthesises around 12,000 – 14,000mg a day (twelve to fourteen grams/day). In fact, multiplied up to human bodyweight, most living beings produce vitamin C in the range of two to fourteen grams a day—even the humble housefly. It is thought human beings lost their ability to synthesise their own vitamin C hundreds of thousands of years ago as part of natural evolutionary change. It is likely that at the time change took place, humans were able to compensate for the loss, because they were living in lush tropical environments in which the natural vitamin C content of food was very high. (In fact the fact it became easily obtainable through diet is probably one of the reasons we stopped synthesising our own vitamin C).

Interestingly, if we work out the vitamin C content of a probable diet eaten by humans at the time changes to our ability to synthesise it took place, it does work out in the two to fourteen gram range. And, as further evidence, allowing for body weight, the present day diet of primates contains a similar daily amount of vitamin C. The recommended daily intake of vitamin C (from food and supplements) in most western countries is sixty milligrams per day. If for a moment we consider the above suggestion about our real optimum need of vitamin C to be correct—then it means we probably obtain some thirty-three to two hundred and thirty times **less** than required for optimal health. Obviously, this could represent a major deficiency.

The present day recommended intake of 60mg per day was arrived at because it represents the amount of vitamin C necessary to prevent scurvy—and at the time it was set, there was no indication the human body required a higher amount. Also, the view that only sixty milligrams a day is required is reinforced by the fact that blood levels of vitamin C will only rise to about 1.5mg per

100ml—no matter how much vitamin C is ingested. It is commonly stated that any amount ingested above the amount needed to raise blood levels to 1.5mg/100ml is excreted in urine, and in effect wasted. But studies do not necessarily confirm this—for instance, at a dose of two grams a day it appears that only about 0.5 grams (25%) is excreted in the urine, the rest being used by the body for various purposes (i.e. 1.44 grams above daily recommended amount of sixty milligrams is utilised by the body in some way).

The body uses vitamin C for a whole range of different functions, many of them directly related to either preventing and/or recovering from cancer. Here is a list of the major roles vitamin C plays in the body:

- Synthesis of collagen, (collagen being one of the major building blocks of the human body).

- Needed by lymphocyte white blood cells for correct functioning of the immune system.

- A general detoxifier—i.e. binding with toxic substances to render them safe.

- An anti-oxidant and free radical scavenger.

- Known to stimulate production of a hyaluronidase inhibitor—a substance used to prevent or retard cancer cell's ability to 'eat their way through body tissues'.

Let's look at how vitamin C can help against cancer in more detail. In their book, Cancer and Vitamin C, Pauling and Cameron examine how cancer patients might live with their illness—as opposed to curing it. For instance, it may be quite possible for an individual to live many years with their cancer; it may be possible to reduce pain, increase appetite as well as influence other factors that contribute to a higher quality of life. Pauling explains that this is not the usual focus of mainstream cancer therapies—rather they usually focus directly on curing cancer which, though worthy, often eclipses or overshadows other therapeutic goals that are just as meaningful and valuable. Modern therapies tend to focus on one particular aspect of cancer tumours—the capacity for proliferation—whereas in fact cancer cells possess two main characteristics. The two main characteristics they possess are as follows:

- The capacity for proliferation—i.e. they grow and divide without restraint.

- The capacity for infiltration—the ability to attack normal tissues and organs—breaking them down to create space for the tumour to grow.

It is the first capacity of tumour cells that has been focussed upon in the search for a cure—and previously, we have examined how chemotherapy compounds target cells as they are dividing. However, Pauling explains that the other capacity possessed by cancer cells—the capacity for infiltration—has largely been ignored. Yet infiltration of organs and tissues is one of the major means by which cancer spreads and causes damage to the body. Surely, he reasoned, 'if this capacity could be targeted, while not eliminating the cancer completely, it might hold it in check for a significant, if not indefinite period of time'.

The mechanism cancer cells use to infiltrate tissues is as follows—cancer cells release two enzymes called hyaluronidase and collagenase. These two enzymes function like mechanical excavators and diggers, dissolving and tearing down tissues surrounding the site of the tumour to create more space for the cancer to grow. Certainly, limiting these enzymes, or limiting the effect they are able to exert against healthy cells, will certainly help slow down the spread of cancer— or even contain it.

The first enzyme, hyaluronidase, directly attacks the intracellular cement between cells. Cells glue themselves tightly together, rather like a line of policemen facing a crowd of rowdy demonstrators need to keep press up tightly to one another. As long as the policemen can stay tight up against each other, they can endure considerable aggression directed towards them—but once their 'line' is breached, protestors may well gain the upper hand. Vitamin C can affect this ability of tumour cells to attack the intracellular cement between cells, because it stimulates production and release of a hyaluronidase inhibitor—in effect helping cells stay tightly 'glued' up against each other.

The second enzyme listed is collagenase. This enzyme has the ability to break apart dense fibres of collagen, directly weakening tissues, bones, cartilage and many other parts of the body. Collagen is the building block of the human body in the same way cellulose is the building block of the plant world—and as mentioned, vitamin C is a major building block of collagen.

Strengthening these natural lines of defence are two ways that vitamin C can help contribute to containing cancer. For instance, one way our body's can deal with cancer is by encapsulating a tumour with a thick impenetrable layer of scar tissue. 'Walling off' a tumour like this means it is contained, restricted in its ability to grow, and unable to release cancer cells into the body. Yet, another way the body protects itself is by 'infiltrating' a tumour with lymphocytes—a type of blood cell that can weaken and eventually destroy cancer cells. For their correct and optimum functioning lymphocytes need adequate stores of vitamin C. (Note: it is often described that a considerable percentage of the weight of a tumour is made up of infiltrating lymphocytes).

An experiment demonstrating the importance of vitamin C to lymphocyte functioning is one where guinea pigs (one of the few animals incapable of synthesising their own vitamin C) were kept on a low vitamin C diet. While on this diet, it was found they would accept skin grafts from other guinea pigs, but as soon as the level of vitamin C in their diet was increased, they immediately began to reject the same skin grafts—i.e. as soon as their lymphocytes regained their natural power and intelligence, they rejected the foreign skin grafts.

Interestingly, it would seem the body manages to successfully deal with cancer more often than it fails. It has been demonstrated from autopsies that cancer is far more prevalent and common than is indicated by cancer statistics—but that it has been effectively dealt with via the mechanisms of lymphocyte infiltration, and 'walling off' behind scar tissue.[76] As Pauling explains in this very important passage:

'The great majority of cancers are held in check by the body; they grow for a while, then regress and disappear, and it is only an occasional one that escapes from control and forms a progressive cancer.'[76]

Pauling put his theories about vitamin C to the test in several animal and human trials—the results of which were extremely positive. In mouse experiments, vitamin C proved effective at delaying the onset of tumours, and in human trails, subjects lived for a considerably longer period of time than controls and experienced very substantial increases in their quality of life. For instance, it was commonly observed that after five to ten days of being on a ten gram per day dose of vitamin C, individuals no longer needed pain-relieving medication.

Individuals in Pauling's trials were reported as having a better appetite, a lifting of spirits, an earlier discharge from hospital and a greater ability to spend their time purposefully. The most important finding, however, was that compared with a matched control group, patients on vitamin C lived substantially longer (an average of ten months longer). Bearing in mind individuals in this trial were late stage terminal cancer cases—i.e. it was felt that nothing more could be done for them—it is interesting to note that 22% of the vitamin C treated patients lived longer than a year, compared to only 0.4% of the control group. Further, some of these 22% went on to live for several years.[77]

The above study was particularly noteworthy because the same doctors and specialists, in the same hospital, treated individuals in both the control group and the vitamin C group. Therefore many of the variables in the study were kept constant (e.g. diet, attitude of professionals, physical surroundings). Another lung cancer study yielded the following results.[78] Of a total of one hundred and twenty-five patients, the following numbers of individuals received the following treatments:

14   Radiation

17   Chemotherapy

24   Vitamin C only

70   No treatment except painkillers

It was surmised that the radiation group contained individuals with a slightly better outlook—this being the reason they were more suitable for radiotherapy treatment. It was considered individuals in the vitamin C group were most comparable with individuals in the 'No treatment group'—in that they were the most advanced cancer cases to which no conventional treatment was offered. The survival rates (in days) of the different groups were as follows:

Radiation   184

Chemotherapy   90

Vitamin C only   187+

No treatment except painkillers   68

These results are obviously very impressive, especially considering they are for lung cancer—one of the more difficult cancers to treat. Note the vitamin C survival rates are the highest of all the treatment modalities, and at the time these results were reported, some of the vitamin C group patients were still living (hence one hundred and eighty-seven days plus). The survival rate of the vitamin C group is twice that of the chemotherapy group, higher than the radiotherapy group, and nearly three times that of the 'no treatment group'. Furthermore, the vitamin C treatment was completely non-toxic, had no side effects, led to a decrease in pain and an improvement in individuals overall quality of life.

Pauling saw in these results, a completely revolutionary way of tackling disease. Rather than using toxic substances with all their debilitating side effects, he saw 'orthomolecular' medicine (i.e. the restoration of proper levels of chemical substances such as vitamins, minerals etc) as holding the promise of defeating and/or controlling disease by strengthening the bodies own natural defence systems. (Mainstream medicine does already use the orthomolecular approach in some instances—for example, the provision of insulin for diabetics.) Pauling viewed vitamin C as a simple and inexpensive treatment suitable for every individual dealing with cancer, regardless of any other treatments they receive. It appears to enhance the action of other treatments, reduce the side effects of toxic medication, and has no deleterious effects on the body—vitamin C is one of the least toxic substances known to man.

A couple of other studies were carried out in Pauling's lifetime and are known as the Moertel or Mayo studies. Unfortunately, in contrast to the positive results Pauling obtained, results obtained in these studies showed no particular benefit for individuals receiving vitamin C. There may, however, be reasons for this—one of which being that in several commentators opinion, these other trials were an orchestrated attempt to discredit Pauling's findings. As a renowned scientist and Nobel Prize winner, Pauling had infuriated the 'cancer establishment' with his claims for vitamin C. At the time the Mayo studies were carried out it was claimed they were identical to the studies carried out by Pauling and Cameron in Scotland. At first glance it does seem as if the Mayo trials were identical, but a more detailed reading shows there were considerable differences. For example, individuals were abruptly taken off vitamin C and placed on chemotherapy if they showed any worsening of subjective factors (i.e. how they felt). This was something Pauling repeatedly warned about, and is something you should be careful of. It is harmful to health to suddenly cease taking a large intake of vitamin C. The reason being that a large intake of vitamin C leads to an increase in the enzymes that process it. If a large intake is suddenly stopped or drastically reduced, the enzymes will scavenge and strip the body of every last bit of vitamin C (this is known as the 'rebound effect'). Because it takes a certain time period for the level of enzymes to reduce down to a more appropriate level, stopping or cutting down a particular intake of vitamin C should be done slowly over a period of a few days.

In the Moertel study only one patient died while on vitamin C, but all the others died soon after their intake of vitamin C was abruptly stopped—possibly because of the shock of the rebound effect. Also, there is question mark over whether individuals in the control group were also taking vitamin C when in terms of the application of correct scientific method, they should not have been. (Urine sample tests detected elevated levels of vitamin C in some control group subjects).

In Pauling's opinion, one of the ironies of conventional care is the continual decreasing of an individual's vitamin C level. It is quite possible that as an individual progresses through a series of treatments, their overall vitamin C level will plummet lower and lower. Let us suppose an individual has a major surgical operation. Eating patterns are likely to be affected for a day or so before and a few days afterwards. This, together with the trauma of surgery (and associated healing), will further lower an individual's vitamin C level. A short while later, the same individual may be given chemotherapy and, once again, vitamin C levels will be placed under further stress. The same applies to radiotherapy. At each stage of conventional care, levels of vitamin C are subjected to stress and end up lower than before the treatment. This is a good reason for individuals receiving conventional therapies to ensure they are always taking an adequate amount of the vitamin.

Using Vitamin C Therapeutically

You may have come across a term often used in relation to vitamin C—bowel tolerance limit. This is the upper limit of oral vitamin C that your bowel will accept. For most people this limit occurs in the eight to thirty grams a day range. The protocol to establish 'bowel tolerance limit' is to start initially with one to two grams per day—spaced out over the day. Intake can then be gradually increased over a number of days, one gram at a time, until you reach your bowel tolerance limit. You will know when you reach your limit because you will start to experience some bloating, gas or diarrhoea (harmless in this context). On reaching this limit you should start to reduce the dosage back down slightly to one that you can take on a sustainable basis (i.e. a dosage where you do not experience gas, bloating or a loosening of stools).

Vitamin C is available in many different forms. The best method of identifying the form that is right for you is to carry out a Metabolic Typing assessment (see p.55)—as each type of vitamin C will have a different effect on your metabolism, depending on which metabolic type you are. However, Linus Pauling regarded ordinary L_Ascorbic Acid as the most suitable form of the vitamin. In their trials, Cameron and Pauling made the vitamin C up into a solution containing the following:

Ascorbic acid	100 grams
Sodium bicarbonate	48 grams
70% Sorbitol syrup	200 millilitres
Distilled water	600 millilitres

Use in the following manner: Take 15ml (one tablespoon = 2.5 grams sodium ascorbate) four times a day after meals. The mixture should be continued indefinitely.[79]

Repeating the guidance given above—you should never suddenly cease taking a high intake of vitamin C but should instead reduce it down gradually over a number of days. It is possible to intake much higher amounts of vitamin C via intravenous drip (e.g. in excess of one hundred grams per day). This will cost more, but is a treatment many alternative cancer clinics include as part of their protocol. If you would like to locate a practitioner offering this therapy see Appendix C: Useful Contacts & Resources (see p.249).

Research indicates vitamin C can work in one of two modes—depending on the amount taken and the route of administration. Taken intravenously in high amounts, it is likely to work as a prooxidant—whereas taken in dry powder form at one to two grams a day, it is likely to work as an antioxidant.

The table below summarises the different methods of using vitamin C, and gives some pointers as to when each method is most useful.

Cost: We estimate the cost of taking one to two grams of vitamin C per day adds up to around £5 ($8) per month (if bought in bulk). Intravenous vitamin C will likely cost you around £60–80 ($96–128) per infusion and needs to be administered by a doctor or nurse.

How to obtain the therapy: You will be able to obtain vitamin C from your local health store. See Appendix C: Useful Contacts & Resources (p.249) for internet sites listing clinics / practitioners who offer intravenous infusion of vitamin C.

Method	Mechanism	Comments
Dry form (1–2 grams per day) used synergistically	Likely to work as an antioxidant	Can form a useful part of an anti-cancer program focussing on oxidative stress reduction (to prevent further DNA damage).
Vitamin C taken orally in solution (e.g. 10g per day)	May work as a prooxidant if trace of iron or copper in the solution.	Pauling obtained very beneficial results with vitamin C in solution in people dealing with 'terminal cancer'.
Intravenous at high dosages (e.g. 120g)	Likely to work as a prooxidant	Reported by many practitioners to be a very useful cancer therapy

Table 18: Summary Of The Different Mechanisms Of Action Of Vitamin C

B

Appendix B:
Important Theories Of Cancer

In this section we shall look at the following theories of cancer:

- Otto Warburg's theory of damaged cell respiration

- Beard's Trophoblast Theory of Cancer

- The B-17 Theory

Though all three theories present themselves as 'a definitive theory of cancer', it is most likely each theory actually reflects *one* of the many faces of the cancer process. Thus we can postulate that each theory is probably true—but not the absolute truth—and should be merged with the others for a more complete 'picture'.

All three theories came into being as a result of the creativity and dedication of their originators. The originators of each theory were dedicated scientists, researchers or doctors, committed to discovering the inner workings of cancer and finding a cure. They are all recognised to be remarkable men, deeply committed to the pursuit of excellence and truth.

We begin with Otto Warburg's Theory of Injured Cell Respiration. Warburg, a man of towering intellectual and scientific ability, was awarded the Nobel Prize twice in his lifetime for his work.

Otto Warburg's Theory of Injured Cell Respiration

Dean Burk, former head of chemistry at the National Cancer Institute, one of the foremost cancer institutions in the world, introduces Otto Warburg as follows:

> 'Otto Warburg won the Nobel Prize in Medicine in 1931 for his discovery of the oxygen-transferring enzyme of cell respiration, and was voted a second Nobel Prize in 1944 for his discovery of the active groups of the hydrogen transferring enzymes. Many universities, like Harvard, Oxford, Heidelberg have offered him honorary degrees. He is a foreign member of the Royal Society in London, a Knight of the Order of Merit founded by Frederick the Great, and was awarded the Great Cross with Star and Shoulder ribbon of the Bundersrepublic. His main interests are Chemistry and Physics of Life. In both fields, no scientists have been more successful.'[80]

As mentioned in the quotation, Warburg is responsible for the discovery of cellular enzymes—in particular, how oxygen and hydrogen are transported in and out of human cells. This work led him to become profoundly interested in both the origin, and the prevention of cancer.

Warburg's theory is based around the fact that human cells have two ways of generating their energy. The first type of energy production is called 'cellular respiration'—which though sounding complex, simply means a cell obtains oxygen from the blood supply and uses it for oxidising (burning) carbohydrates. In effect, a cell keeps a small bonfire burning inside itself—and the 'fire' needs to remain fully alight for the cell to remain healthy. For the fire to remain alight, the cells' oxygen-transferring mechanism (i.e. the enzymes that transfer oxygen from outside to inside the cell) must be fully functional, and sufficient oxygen must be available in the blood stream.

The analogy of a fire burning inside a cell is useful to consider further. For just as a fire can be dampened down, and eventually extinguished by placing a thick sheet over it, so human cells are deeply affected when they cannot obtain sufficient oxygen to keep their own 'fire' burning. If this ever happens, and there is a risk of a 'power cut', cells switch over to another method of generating their energy—energy by fermentation. This means a cell stops using oxygen to generate its energy, and starts fermenting glucose into lactic acid, roughly the same way that yeast turns sugary water into wine.

Though a failsafe mechanism (i.e. a back-up generator), the generation of energy via fermentation of glucose causes several serious problems for human beings. First, energy production via fermentation is inefficient compared with cellular oxygen respiration—more fuel is used, but there is less energy output. Also fermentation produces large quantities of lactic acid waste, which the liver has to recycle back into glucose. This can mean the liver ends up dong a lot of work for cells which are using fermentation to generate their energy.

Further, the amount of energy commonly generated via fermentation is around one hundred times less than the amount of energy generated via cellular respiration. The first impact of this drop in energy could be cellular death—as a cell might not have enough energy to survive. Ironically, this is preferable because at least the cell is prevented from becoming 'cancerous'. Warburg explains the danger of cancer arises from a cell trying to perform all of its normal functions on the limited energy generated from fermentation.

This is because by switching itself over to fermentation the cell has, in effect, 'switched' itself back in time—back to a primitive era. The use of fermentation within a cell corresponds to a period in evolution billions of years ago—the time when single celled beings developed. The problem, however, is cells at this early stage of evolution (e.g. algae and other 'primitive' life forms) lack the controls that limit cell division and growth. Rather, they keep dividing and multiplying without cessation. Take the example of yeast—during the production of wine, yeast cells keep multiplying until they have either metabolised all the sugar, or poisoned themselves in their waste (alcohol).

If human cells begin functioning like this we call it cancer, and Warburg describes this transition from cellular respiration to fermentation as a transition from heaven to hell. Heaven to hell because complex life forms (i.e. humans) are founded upon fully functioning cellular oxygen respiration. Only 'primitive' life forms can survive long-term using fermentation to generate their energy.

As well as losing their 'regulatory' controls, when cells switch over to fermentation they lose their ability to 'differentiate'. The term 'differentiate' sounds complex, but it just means cells can become different. For instance, looking at your hand, it is made up of cells which have become fingernail growing cells, cells which have become skin cells, etc—all working together in perfect harmony. Differentiation is something that belongs to higher forms of life as it allows far greater complexity of physical being. In contrast, a tumour is an area where 'differentiation' has broken down. Rather than cells 'maturing' and taking on a specialised form that helps the complex whole, they remain 'immature', more similar and form an amorphous mass.

Warburg questions the link between the failure of oxygen metabolism (cellular respiration) and the breakdown of differentiation—and asks why the two are linked. The answer he provides is interesting.

In comparison with cellular respiration, fermentation is a far simpler process with fewer steps needed to complete it. Comparing them, both follow the same first four steps, but then fermentation only needs one additional step to reach its final goal (lactic acid)—whereas cellular respiration needs an additional thirty steps to reach its end point. Therefore it is the complexity of cellular respiration which supports differentiation—and the complexity of our species.

It can be likened to a modern day oil refinery. Oil goes in one end and goes through an enormous series of different reactions, with different chemicals and products extracted at various stages in the process. The complexity of such a plant can be seen in the vast array of interconnecting pipes and tubes that form the classic picture of an oil refinery. In the same way as the complexity of the oil refinery and its products support global civilization, the complexity of oxygen metabolism support and maintain the incredible complexity of the human body. Warburg poetically expresses the situation:

> 'When [cellular] respiration disappears, life does not disappear, but the meaning of life disappears, and what remains are growing machines that destroy the body in which they grow.'[81]

Warburg points out that even the yeast cell, one of life's simplest cells, cannot maintain its structure by fermentation alone:

> '…it degenerates into bizarre forms. However as Pasteur showed, it is rejuvenated in a wonderful manner if it comes into contact with oxygen for a short time.'[82]

Therefore how much more does absence of cellular respiration and the resultant increase in fermentation affect our more complex human structure? Another way of describing the role cellular respiration plays is the concept of a 'forced steady state'.

'Forced steady state' in this context refers to the 'invisible' work cellular respiration does in maintaining the complexity of life. An analogy is a ball held in place at the top of an incline by an invisible force. When the ball is at the top of the incline, our complex bodies function perfectly. The 'invisible force' that keeps the ball at the top of the incline corresponds to the 'work' being done by cellular respiration. However, as soon as cells switch over to fermentation, the invisible 'work' being done by cellular respiration vanishes—and the ball rolls down the incline to the bottom—to the level of de-differentiation and cancer.

To summarise what we have described about the properties of cells when they become cancerous, three factors that describe a tumour are:

- It has a high fermentation index—the greater the level of fermentation the higher the malignancy

- It lacks any regulation of growth and its cells keep dividing

- It is a de-differentiated amorphous mass

What causes damage to cellular respiration?

In short, what Warburg calls 'respiratory poisons'. These can be any substance ingested, breathed or which we are exposed to, that injure cells' cellular respiration mechanisms. Numerous chemicals in pollution and smoke, as well as many other 'unnatural ingredients' of modern life, are respiratory poisons.

A cell doesn't switch totally over from one mode to the other in one step. Rather, at first cellular respiration may be only slightly damaged—for example the ratio of cellular respiration to fermentation energy production might become 99:1. Then a time later, further damage might leave the ratio at 90:1—and so on. Though maybe unnoticeable for many years, the groundwork is being laid for cancer.

Three factors which can contribute to increasing fermentation within a cell are:

- Further injury to the cellular respiration components by 'respiratory poisons' in food, air or water (e.g. pesticides and food additives).

- Further lowering of oxygen supply to cells (e.g. further degrading of blood supply)

- Cellular strain caused by neighbours who have already switched over to fermentation.

Warburg's recommendations for ensuring we do not contract cancer—and as a therapy if we have already done so—is to do everything possible to re-establish an environment conducive to efficient cellular respiration. Steps towards this should include:

- Cleaning our environment of all respiratory poisons (carcinogenic toxins).

- Supplementation of diet with vitamins and other nutrient factors that work together with the cell in supplying it with oxygen.

- Exercise to keep the blood flowing through all the body's tissues (to ensure adequate supply of oxygen to cells).

- Use of therapies that oxygenate the body and/or stimulate the oxidative processes within cells (e.g. ozone therapy).

Final Points

Warburg's ideas form an impressive and grand theory of cancer. It provides insights into many important processes, as well as indicating where therapeutic efforts might be directed. Also it ties in very well with actual practical aspects of the disease. For instance, it is true that the degree of fermentation present in a tumour is an indication of its virulence. Also, the enormous need of cancer cells for glucose and the resulting strain placed on the liver (to process lactic acid back into glucose) is reflected in the wasting diseases experienced by so many individuals with cancer (cachexia).

Warburg's theory is based on some very simple and ingenious experiments he devised. It is worth briefly mentioning these because they offer some proof of Warburg's theories. The first experiment used a very simple piece of apparatus that enabled cells to be cultured with a controllable atmosphere of oxygen around them. Using this apparatus, Warburg demonstrated that if the oxygen level was reduced until the cells cellular respiration was inhibited by 35% for forty-eight hours, ensuing cell lines started to move towards cancerous cells (within two cell divisions). Warburg mentions that 'oxygen pressures' that inhibit respiration by 35% can occur at the end of blood capillaries in living animals'—(hence his recommendation for good exercise).[83]

The second experiment involved injecting tetanus spores into mice. Tetanus spores were used because they only incubate to maturity in low oxygen conditions. Spores were injected into three types of mice—healthy mice, pregnant mice and mice with cancerous growths. The results were as follows: The tetanus spores did not incubate in the first two groups of mice (healthy and pregnant), but did germinate in the mice with tumours. This demonstrated that mice with tumours had a low oxygen environment in their body (or the spores would not have germinated).

The last words of this section rightfully go to Otto Warburg himself:

> 'Nobody today can say that one does not know what cancer and its prime cause be. On the contrary, there is no disease whose prime cause is better known, so that today ignorance is no longer an excuse that one cannot do more about prevention. That prevention of cancer will come there is no doubt, for man wishes to survive. But how long prevention will be avoided depends on how long the prophets of agnosticism [scepticism] will succeed in inhibiting the application of scientific knowledge in the cancer field. In the meantime, millions of men must die of cancer unnecessarily.'

Beard's Trophoblast Theory of Cancer

John Beard's Trophoblast Theory is another well worked out theory of cancer. Furthermore, the foundations of the theory have been confirmed by recent research—which is remarkable considering Beard elaborated the theory over one hundred years ago. In the course of his work, Beard noticed a link between development of cancer in the human foetus (on or shortly after the 56th day of pregnancy) and the abnormal development of the foetus's pancreas. This observation inspired in him the 'Trophoblast Theory of Cancer'.

Trophoblast cells are very closely related to stem cells. We discussed stem cells earlier in relation to bone marrow transplants—they are cells that, when stimulated by an appropriate stimulus, transform themselves into any type of cell required in the human body. Specifically, when stimulated by the hormone oestrogen they become Trophoblast cells otherwise known as 'Healing Cells'. Trophoblast cells or 'Healing Cells' are employed at two particular times— either as part of a healing process to repair the body, or at conception, for carving out a niche for the embryo to attach itself to the uterine wall.

The Trophoblast Theory of Cancer explains that cancer occurs when Trophoblast cells are not correctly terminated after they have completed their assigned healing function. Instead they continue 'healing'—but they have now become 'cancerous' because rather than performing a useful role, their 'healing activity' causes havoc in the body (i.e. cancer tumours). A further complication is caused because Trophoblast cells are natural host cells (i.e. not intruders) and therefore the body doesn't recognise them as dangerous and, even though they have become cancerous, leaves them alone.

Obviously the dangers of a Trophoblast cell not being correctly terminated are serious—so what is the mechanism the body uses to ensure the action of trophoblasts are correctly terminated? Remarkably—and this is the link with the pancreas—enzymes such as chymotrypsin are synthesised by the pancreas and released into the blood stream. These circulate in the blood and 'eat' through the outer protein layer of any Trophoblast cells they encounter (enzymes 'digest' proteins). As soon as the Trophoblasts outer layer of protein (along with the antigens that identify it as a host cell) have been 'eaten' away, its camouflage is compromised and it is rendered vulnerable to destruction by the immune system.

Going back to the abnormal development of cancer in the foetus—cancer is observed to occur in the foetus whose pancreas has not properly developed by the 56th day—and therefore has not started releasing chymotrypsin enzyme into the bloodstream. The cancer that occurs to mother and baby when this happens is known as chorionepithelioma, and is considered to be one of the most malignant of all cancers. Likewise, there is the same risk of cancer in an adult or a child if the pancreas is not releasing sufficient enzymes into the bloodstream and so ensuring the 'healing' activity of Trophoblasts is halted at the correct time.

Further evidence of the close relationship of healing to cancer is provided by the fact that if tissue taken from a wound is given to a histopathologist (professional in the microscopic structure of tissue), most likely they would not be able to determine whether the tissue sample had been taken from a wound undergoing healing, or a cancerous tumour.[84] In addition, it is not uncommon to read case reports where cancer follows soon after a major injury such as a broken arm or leg.

A very interesting implication of the Beardian theory relates to testing for cancer. In line with the Beardian theory, the presence of cancer should be able to be detected with a more sensitive version of a common pregnancy testing kit, rather than with biopsies (which carry the risk of releasing cancer cells into the body). The reason is that after a stem cell has been stimulated by oestrogen hormone to become a Trophoblast cell, the Trophoblast cell releases its own hormone called chorionic gonadotrophin (hCG). Day writes:

> '[This hormone] can be detected in urine with a simple test that is 92% accurate in all cases. In regard to a positive test result, Griffin notes: 'If the patient is a woman, she is either pregnant or has cancer. If he is a man, cancer can be the only cause'. Yet the medical industry, in full possession and knowledge of this information and associated tests, still insists on recommending dangerous biopsy operations to detect cancerous growths, the biopsies themselves sometimes contributing to the spread of cancer cells through the body when cuts in the tumours are made.'[85]

In terms of confirming whether the above is true, because cancer cells are Trophoblast cells (either created during the initial phase of pregnancy, or as a part of a healing process) it should be possible to test for the presence of the hormone chorionic gonadotrophin (hCG) in individuals with various cancers. If this were shown to be true, it would go a long way in confirming John Beard's theory.

In 1995, such evidence was provided. Ralph Moss writes:

> 'In mid-1995, Prof. Hernan Acevedo and colleagues showed that the 'synthesis and statement of hCG…is a common biochemical denominator of cancer'. Acevedo demonstrated the presence of hCG, its subunits, and/or fragments, in eighty-five different cancer cell lines. He also consistently found hCG in human malignant tumour tissues.

Acevedo concluded that 'hCG the hormone of pregnancy and development that also has chemical and physiological properties of growth factors, is a common phenotype characteristic of cancer'. In his 1995 article in the journal Cancer, Acevedo concluded that, after nearly a century, 'Beard has been proven to be conceptually correct...'[86]

A cancer hCG test needs to be far more sensitive than a normal pharmacy shop pregnancy test to pick up the presence of cancer, though of course they measure and detect the same hormone. See the end of this section for details of where an hCG test can be carried out.

As has been described, in the Beardian cancer theory pancreatic enzymes play an important role in the body. There are three broad strategies commonly expounded by unconventional cancer professionals to ensure that levels remain high (note that some contradict each other).

1   Supplement enzymes in the diet.

2   Eat fresh organic foods—preferably vegetables, as the process of digesting meat uses significant amounts of enzymes. (The body needs to utilize far more enzymes digesting meat than when it digests vegetable matter because proteins are far more difficult than carbohydrates to separate and break into individual component parts)

3   Third is the recommendation made by Metabolic Typing, that for optimum pancreas functioning, the biochemistry of food eaten should match an individual's unique requirements. In Metabolic Typing terminology this might mean that a high protein, fat & oil based diet might meet an individuals requirements better than a carbohydrate based diet (and vice-versa).

In summary, we can say that Beard's ideas about the cause of cancer are interesting and provocative. Provocative in the sense that Beard's observations tie in with much of what happens in 'reality' during cancer, but at the same time suggest a cause (enzyme deficiency) that is quite unacceptable to most mainstream cancer institutions at the present time. Further, Beard's observation, over one hundred years ago, of the link between the abnormal development of the pancreas and the development of cancer, is a very significant insight—and for this reason alone the theory deserves far more attention than it has received. It is of note that Moss considers the Beardian theory to be 'the theory' of cancer most likely to be 'true' (see p.167). Results of an 'authorised' enzyme study, examining the effect enzymes exert on cancer are due in the next few years.[87] The results are looked forward to with anticipation.

Availability Of The HCG Hormone Test:

This is the only channel we know of, but a local lab in your area may be offering the test.

Name: The Navarro beta-HCG urine cancer test—a safe, cost-effective, non-invasive, accurate screening test for Cancer.

Proceedure: Send urine samples by mail to Dr. Efren F. Navarro

The specimen should be the first urine after midnight. For women, there should be no sexual contact for 12 days before collecting the urine specimen. Do not send a urine sample of a woman who is pregnant. For men, there should be no sexual contact for 18-24 hours before the sample is taken.

Directions:

a) Mix 50cc of urine with 200cc of acetone (can be purchased from hardware store or pharmacy) and 5cc of 70% isopropyl rubbing alcohol or 95% ethyl alcohol. Stir and mix well.

b) Let the mixture stand for 2 hours in refrigerator until a sediment forms.

c) Throw off about half of the urine-acetone mixture without losing any sediments. Filter the remaining mixture through a coffee filter paper or a laboratory filter paper to retain the sediment.

d) After filtration, air dry the filter paper with the sediments.

e) Fold the filter and place it in a plastic bag.

If the results are wanted quickly, send the specimen by courier (FedEx, UPS, or DHL) or by USPS Global Priority Mail to Dr. Navarro together with the patient's name, age, sex, brief medical history and/or diagnosis, and a Xerox copy of a money order or check for $45, made out to Erlinda N. Suarez. Otherwise, send the specimen by regular airmail and allow 4-6 weeks for test result delivery.

Dr. Navarro's address is:

Dr. Efren F. Navarro, M.D.
3553 Sining Street
Morningside Terrace
Santa Mesa, Manila 2806
Philippines

☎: 011 632-714-7442
Email: efnavmed@compass.com.ph

Mail the money order or check (personal checks drawn on a U.S. bank are also acceptable) to:

Ms. Erlinda N. Suarez
631 Peregrine Drive

Palatine, IL 60067-7005

The specimen will be tested immediately upon arrival and the results sent by email as soon as they become available to the patient's and/or physician's email address. The official report will be sent back by airmail.

The B-17 Hypothesis

B-17 is probably one of the most controversial of all conventional and alternative cancer therapies. There have been several studies that have shown its efficacy in animals, and many doctors attest to its powers of healing and also its value as a palliative agent (though no noteworthy human studies have been carried out). However, it is worth emphasising from the beginning that, in therapeutic terms, the main benefit clinically reported from the use of B-17 is in regard to the prevention of secondary cancer (metastases), and then only when it is used in very large dosages.

It is also worth clarifying that B-17 is also known as amygdalin or laetrile. The difference between the three is as follows—amygdalin is the name of the chemical substance found in nature. Laetrile is the synthetic version of the compound, and B-17 is the name given by Dean Burke (of the National Cancer Institute), in recognition of its value to the human body i.e. he classified it as the 17th B vitamin (a vitamin being a vital substance the body needs to obtain from the outside, as it cannot manufacture it itself).

The B-17 story begins with anthropological studies looking into the health of various populations. Studies identified several groups who experience a 'higher' level of health than is commonly experienced by others. 'Good health' here means longevity, freedom from disease, good teeth, physical stamina into old age etc. One culture identified was the Hunzas who live in a mountainous region in Northern India (Kashmir region). People in this culture commonly live to ages well over a hundred, as well as maintain a high level of physical strength and stamina into advanced age. At the time of the studies, cancer was completely unknown in the Hunza culture—and it was reported individuals lived completely free of the fear and experience of cancer.

After identifying groups of people who experience a higher level of health, studies proceeded to identify particular factors responsible for each group's increased health and fitness. Many obvious factors were identified, such as freedom from processed foods, drinking fresh uncontaminated mineral rich water, fresh unpolluted air etc. However, one not so obvious factor was identified—the inclusion in their diets of bitter substances, quite common in nature, called nitrilosides.

The inclusion of bitter substances in the diet was particularly well reflected in the Hunza culture. In the Hunza culture, apricots play a very important role. They are used in cooking (as an oil), they are included in the ingredients for makeup and other 'personal care products', and when the actual apricots are eaten (fresh or dried daily), they are always eaten along with the apricot kernel (which is released when the nut is cracked open).

After the high rate of consumption of nitrilosides was observed, research focussed on the role these compounds play in the body. Research identified that apricot kernels contain an active substance which, as described above, is called amygdalin. Amygdalin is extremely bitter and though found in many types of fruit, vegetables, nuts and seeds, it is only in very small quantities compared with the apricot kernel. Apple seeds are the food that contains the next greatest amount (which is, some B-17 advocates suggest, the source and the original meaning of the proverb, 'An apple a day keeps the doctor away').

Amygdalin turns out to be a substance that plays a most unusual role in the body. Strange as it may seem, in terms of being healthy, amygdalin partly consists of a cyanide molecule, safely locked up inside two harmless glucose molecules. (Note: B-12 is also a cyanide molecule, hence the chemical name for B-12 of *cyano*cobalamin). Because the cyanide molecule is securely locked up, and only a special key can open it, it is non-toxic if eaten (on its own) because normal cells of the body do not contain (in any significant amount) the special key needed to open the 'chemical safe' and release the cyanide molecule. Some critics still claim that if it contains cyanide it must be dangerous. But the fact is the cyanide is bound tightly and securely with the glucose molecules and can only be released by the appropriate 'key'. And, as mentioned above, B-12 is an example of another essential cyanide molecule.

For proof of amygdalin's safety it is possible to cite a number of animal studies that looked at the health of animals fed extremely large dosages of the chemical, often for a period of years. No dangerous or worrying side effects were identified in any of the studies. The only side effect was sleepiness in a sheep fed huge dosages of the chemical. However, the sheep soon recovered its alertness after the dose was lowered.[88] Of course, the mention of cyanide conjures up images of the Nazi gas chambers. It is important to point out that a particular

Disease	Prevented by	Death Rate(*)	Status
Scurvy	Vitamin C (ascorbic)	varies	Defeated
Pellagra	Vitamin B3 (niacin)	97%	Defeated
P.Anemia	Vitamin B12 (+ folic acid)	99%	Defeated
Beriberi	Vitamin B1 (thiamine)		Defeated
Cancer	Vitamin B17 (laetrile)	varies	Defeated?
(*) Expected mortality rate at the time, once diagnosed			

Table 19: Metabolic Diseases[93]

form of man-made cyanide called potassium cyanide was used in the death camps, not amygdalin.

In terms of the chemistry of the amygdalin molecule, the cyanide—present in the form of hydrocyanic acid—can be unlocked from the glucose molecules by only one particular enzyme. This enzyme is called Glucosidase. By strange coincidence it is estimated there is over three thousand times more Glucosidase present in a cancer cell than in healthy cells.[89] This means, as B-17 is circulating around the body, if it happens upon a cancer cell, then the Glucosidase present in the cancer cell unlocks the B-17 molecule, releases the cyanide and turns it into hydrogen cyanide. The hydrogen cyanide, because it has been released exactly at the target site, poisons and kills the cancer cell.

It is the Glucosidase in the cancer cell that is the most important step in the process. Hydrocyanic acid, the form of the cyanide when it is locked up in the B-17 molecule, is a harmless substance and is widely present in low amounts in the seeds of many common fruits. The Glucosidase, though, turns the hydrocyanic acid into hydrogen cyanide and creates a powerful cancer-cell-killing toxin.

Nature has more up her sleeve. The B-17 molecule also contains benzaldehyde, another cancer-cell-killing chemical. Again the benzaldehyde is only released by the unlocking enzyme present in the cancer cell. Benzaldehyde has been employed by chemotherapists and shows significant anti-tumour activity as well as an ability to 'de-transform' malignant cells (i.e. turn them back to normal—dedifferentiate).xc Reporting on a study of benzaldehyde, the authors state, 'the overall objective response rate was fifty-five percent…''seven patients achieved complete response, twenty-nine achieved partial response, twenty-four remained stable, and five showed progressive disease'.[91]

In completing its response to B-17, the body has mechanisms to deal with any free cyanide. Free hydrogen cyanide gets converted into Thiocyanate, a useful substance that the body uses to regulate blood pressure, and manufacture B-12. The conversion of free cyanide into thiocyanate is carried out via another enzyme called rhodenase, widely present in healthy cells. Also any free benzaldehyde gets converted into benzoic acid, another useful substance that is an analgesic and an antiseptic.

As you can appreciate, the action of B-17 seems almost too perfect to be an accident, and this is why Dean Burk, head of chemistry at the National Cancer Institute, along with other researchers, gave it the designation as the seventeenth B vitamin. B-17 is literally the anti-cancer vitamin. Earlier we described nitrilosides, and apricot kernels in particular, as bitter tasting. This is a point of great interest and B-17 advocates point out that our modern day western diet is almost completely devoid of bitter foods. In contrast, many of the foods consumed are sweet or salty and we have completely lost the taste for 'bitterness'. We tend to view bitter foods as unpleasant tasting even though 'bitterness' is one of the prime 'senses' of the tongue.

B-17 advocates claim that the present day epidemic of cancer is related to our overwhelmingly sweet, salty and highly processed diet lacking in bitter foods. They point to what they consider a historical analogy—the illness of scurvy. Scurvy was an illness that sailors used to particularly fear. And for good reason: between 1600 and 1800 over one million British sailors died of this illness.[92] However it is documented that a cure (consuming foods with high vitamin C content) had already been discovered for this illness in 1535. However it wasn't until 1795—some two hundred and sixty years after the first documented knowledge of a cure—that the relevant 'authorities' accepted vitamin C both prevents and cures scurvy. It took nearly three hundred years of unnecessary suffering and death before authorities were willing to accept the evidence. Moreover, scurvy is not the only historical example of a devastating illness found (after considerable time) to be easily curable by specific nutrients. Day lists the following table of illnesses that have ravaged whole populations before it was recognised that they were in fact simple deficiency illnesses.

The table provocatively lists cancer and questions whether it has already been defeated. Though in our view a serious overstatement, the B-17 Theory of Cancer certainly illuminates some valuable areas for future research. Research carried out so far has produced some reasonably positive results—though as yet, only animal studies have been carried out.

Studies carried out on B-17

We will quote Day extensively in his summary of studies. He writes:

> 'The National Cancer Institutes Dr Dean Burk oversaw many of the details surrounding the testing of laetrile in the 1970's. Burk states that positive, statistically highly significant, anti-cancer activity by laetrile in animal tumour systems has been observed in at least five independent institutions in three widely separated countries of the world, with a variety of animal cancers:[94]
>
> Southern Research Institute (Birmingham Alabama), for the NCI. [Increase,] ... in a majority of two hundred and eighty BDF1 mice bearing Lewis lung cancers, treated with up to 400mg Laetrile per Kg body weight, with respect to increased median life span (3rd December 1973).
>
> Sloan Kettering (New York) with two hundred and eighty CD8 F1 mice bearing spontaneous mammary carcinomas, inhibition of

formation of lung metastases, inhibition of growth of primary tumours, and greater health and appearance of animal hosts, upon treatment with 1–2gm Laetrile/pre Kg body weight/day (13 June 1973).

Scind Laboratories, University of San Francisco, four hundred rats bearing Walker two hundred and fifty-six carcinoma (two hundred treated with Amygdalin, two hundred controls), with 80% increase in lifespan at optimum dosage (500mg Amygdalin/Kg body weight) (10th October 1968).

NCI Director Carl Baker wrote to the Congressman Edwin W Edwards on 26th January 1971: "The data provided by the McNaughton Foundation certainly indicates some activity in animal tumour systems."

Pasteur Institute (Paris), with human cancer strain maintained in mice, treated at optimal dosage of 500mg Amygdalin…kg body weight/day, increased lifespan and delayed tumour growth up to 100% (6th December 1971)

Institute Von Ardenne (Dresden, Germany), H strain mice bearing Ehrlich ascites carcinoma treated with bitter almond amygdalin ad libitum in addition to regular chow diet, yielded increased lifespan and decreased rate of cancer growth, treatment beginning fifteen days before cancer inoculation (arch Geschwulstorsch. 42, 135–7 (1973)).

As you may have noticed, one of the difficulties of using B-17 would seem to be the high levels that are required for therapeutic effect—the concentrations listed above are very high (e.g. 500mg/kg body weight). This means therapy is best carried using intravenous infusion. A doctor who has extensive experience of using laetrile (synthetic form of B-17), especially with terminal cancer cases, is Dr Ernesto Contreras. Dr Contreras has been running his clinic in Mexico for over thirty years. His utilisation of Laetrile is always in conjunction with wide ranging nutritional and detoxification support, specifically, high levels of enzymes and vitamin A. About laetrile Dr Contreras writes:

> 'The palliative action [i.e. improved comfort] is in about 60% of the cases. Frequently, enough to be significant, I see arrest of the disease or even regression in some 15% of the very advanced cases.'[95]

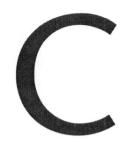

Appendix C:
Useful Contacts & Resources

Useful contacts

Please see www.cancure.org/directory_clinics.htm for a comprehensive listing of unconventional cancer treatment clinics around the world.

Cancer Options is a private, cancer consultancy where you can obtain consultancy, research and coaching for all the different cancer treatments and therapies.

Cancer Options Ltd
10 Harley Street
London
WIG 9PF
United Kingdom

Tel/Fax +44(0) 845 009 2041
Site: www.canceroptions.co.uk
Email: enquiries@canceroptions.co.uk

Brackendene Clinic, run by Dr Paul Wayman offers various unconventional/ complementary therapies including a version of metabolic therapy and intravenous B-17.

Brackendene Clinic
10 Copse Road
Venwood, Dorset
BH31 6HB
England

☎: 01202 824109
🕿: 01202 820739

Etienne Callebout, M.D offers a wide variety of unconventional therapies including 714X, aloe vera, B-17, bovine cartilage, DMSO, Wobe-Mugos and other enzymes, glandulars, green tea, Iscador, flaxseed oil, Maitake mushrooms, cancer vaccines, shark cartilage, and other homeopathic and herbal remedies.

Etienne Callebout, M.D
10 Harley Street
London
England
W1N1AA

☎: 0207 2 55 2232
☎: 07930 336348
🕿: 01582 769832

Munro-Hall Clinic run by Dr. G. Munro-Hall BDS, FIAOMT and Dr. L. Munro-Hall BDS specialise in holistic dentistry but also offer a detox program that can include intravenous infusions of vitamins and B-17.

Wick End Farm
Wick End
Stagsden
Beds
MK43 8TS
England

Tel 07050-611333
Fax 07050-611444

The Chiron Clinic run by Dr. Nyjon Eccles offers several treatments useful for individuals dealing with cancer including. For men and women with breast cancer and/or who are interested in screening The Chiron Clinic offer thermal imaging. See their website for more details.

The Chiron Clinic
121 Harley Street
London
W1G 6AX

☎: +44 (0)20 7224 4622
🖷: +44 (0)20 7224 4655
E-mail Info@ChironClinic.com
Web: www.chironclinic.com

Information sites:

Centre for Advancement in Cancer Education: A non-profit cancer information, counselling and referral agency
>Site: www.beatcancer.org

Ralph Moss's guide to cancer therapy centres of excellence
>Site: www.clinicsofexcellence.com

Center for Advancement in Cancer Education
>Site: www.beatcancer.org

Life Extension Foundation
>Site: www.lef.org

WHALE: Includes practitioner listing, articles, interviews, etc.
>Site: www.whale.to

Cancer Cure Foundation: Therapies, personal experiences, etc
>Site: www.cancure.org

Life Extension Foundation: Cancer protocols, supplements, research.
>Site: www.lef.org

Warburg's Prime Cause of Cancer Lecture:
>Site: www.ozonetherapy.co.uk/warburg.htm

Glutathione resources:

Studies: http://members.shaw.ca/duncancrow/medline_links.html

Whey protein & cancer:
>http://members.shaw.ca/widewest/WPC-as-a-Cysteine-Donor.pdf

Dr. Gutman's ebook on Glutathione:

>   http://members.shaw.ca/widewest/GSH_ebook.zip

Philip Day's website covering a variety of health issues:

>   Site: www.credence.org

The Annie Appleseed Project

>   Site: www.annieappleseedproject.org

Additional Resources for the John Boik Section:

Most of the compounds that Boik discusses are easily available. However some are only just coming into production as standardised extracts or pure formulations. Here is some pointers for the more difficult to locate substances:

- Luteolin: www.lutimax.com/order.html

- Asiatic acid: www.bnatural-online.com

- CAPE (use raw propolis): www.apitherapy.biz

- Standardized Astragalus (70% polysaccharides): www.solgar.com

- Arctigenin: www.kingherb.com

- Apigenin: Not common commercially—but see www.iherb.com/neurodef.html for a mix which provides a considerable daily quantity.

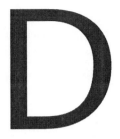

Appendix D: Natural Compounds Against Cancer Costings

In this appendix we will work through costings associated with the compounds outlined earlier in the section 'Natural Anti-Cancer Compounds Discussed By John Boik'. In the following pages we include three tables. The first, outlines costs associated with each of the compounds discussed by Boik (and for each compound we have indicated a cost for a particular dose—usually at the lower end of the suggested dosage guideline).

The second table illustrates a scenario, whereby the suggested numbers of compounds are selected from each group (e.g. 1 of 2, or 2 of 4, etc), to work out an illustrative cost. Our total comes to £15.66 ($25.06) per day—though of course this is only a rough figure, and one based on the dosage we have chosen for each compound. We should note, we have not always chosen the lowest cost compound(s) from each group. In the third table—for all compounds except arctigenin (arctigenin is not yet commercially available)—we have listed a supplier. You will note that all the suppliers are based in the US. We have used

US companies because their products are usually cheaper, and they tend to hold a wider range of stock. However, in many cases you will be able to locate a supplier in your country. To make the tables less cluttered—we have left all the prices in dollars. (Note Asiatic acid & Geraniol are also unavailable in *high percentage* standardised extracts).

It is important to reiterate, that the dosage recommendations are preliminary, and for research purposes only. This is an evolving field, and there is a lot more research needing to be carried out. It is important to work with a medical practitioner, especially as you will need careful monitoring when taking some of the compounds listed (e.g. vitamin A & D3). With all the compounds, start with a low dose and watch for possible adverse reactions. If you note any reactions, stop that particular compound immediately. For more in-depth descriptions of each compound and its 'method of action', please see John Boik's excellent book, 'Natural Compounds in Cancer Therapy'.

Choice	Compound	Research Indicated Range	Example dose cost / day
Direct Acting Compounds (Compounds that Act directly upon cancer cells)			
2 of 4	Apigenin	0.1 – 0.6 g per day	$0.50 / 100 mg
	Luteolin	0.17 – 1.8 g per day	$2.00 / 200 mg
	Genistein	0.1 – 1.1 g per day	$0.60 / 670 mg
	Quercetin	0.25 – 1.8 g per day	$0.18 / 500 mg
1 of 2	Arctigenin	0.65 g per day	Not readily available
	Arctium seed	12 g per day	$0.86 / 12 grams
1 of 2	Boswellic acid	1.8 g per day	$0.98 / 1.8 grams
	Asiatic acid	1.7 g per day	Not readily available
1 of 1	CAPE	3 – 15 g per day	$1.50 / 10g bee propolis
1 of 1	Curcumin	1.5 – 1.8 g per day	$0.62 / 1.5 g
1 of 1	Emodin	0.16 – 0.81g per day	$1.60 / 160mg
1 of 1	EPA/DHA	6 – 21 g per day	$0.33 / 6 grams
0 or 1	Garlic	6 – 15 g per day	$0.64 / 6 gram
1 of 3	Limonene	7.3 – 14 g per day	$3.14 / 7.3 gram
	Perillyl alcohol	1.3 – 9 g per day	$1.70 / 1.3 gram
	Geraniol	0.27 – 5.7 g per day	Lavender oil for low amt.
1 of 1	Parthenolide	17 mg per day	$0.65 / 17 mg
1 of 1	Resveratrol	68 – 410 mg per day	320mg from Emodin mix
1 of 1	Selenium	250–1100µg per day	$0.15 / 400 µg
1 of 1	Vit. A emulsified	50000–600000 i.u.	$0.08 / 50,000 i.u.
1 of 1	Vit. (1,25-D3)	0.75–2.5 µg per day	$1.86/0.75µg – Rocaltrol
1 of 2	Vitamin E	440–1700 i.u per day	$0.27 / 1000 i.u.
	Vitamin E succinate	440–1700 i.u per day	$0.25 / 800 i.u.
Indirect-Acting Compounds (action by influencing the cancer cells environment)			
1 of 2	Anthocyanidins	0.12 – 1.8 g per day	$1.03 / 120 mg
	Proanthocyanidins	0.49 – 1.8 g per day	$1.60 / 490 mg
1 of 2	Ruscogenins	100 – 130 mg per day	$1.40 / 40mg
	Aesin extract	150 mg per day	160mg inc. in cell above
0 or 1	Vitamin C	1 – 2 g per day	$0.15 / 2 grams
Immune Stimulants (compounds that enhance the immune system)			
1 of 1	Bromelain	1 – 4 g per day	$1.05 / 3.5 grams
1 of 1	Astragalus	Inc. in PSP/PSK grp	$1.50 /=30g in decoction
1 of 2	Siberian ginseng	Inc. in PSP/PSK grp	$0.33 /= 12g in decoction
	Ginsenoside (Panax)	110 - 340mg	$0.57 / 110 mg
1 of 3	PSP/PSK (Coliolus)	2–9g polysaccharides /day. (Approx 7% of raw product)	$1.50 / 3 gram extract
	Ganoderma		$0.90 / 1.9 gram extract
	Shiitake		$0.60 / 450mg extract
1 of 1	Melatonin	3 – 20 mg per day	$0.35 / 10 mg
0 or 1	Glutamine	8 – 30 per day	$1.76 / 8 gram
Compounds For Which The Required Dose Is Relatively Uncertain			
0 of 3	EGCG	0.46 – 0.55 g per day	$0.68 / 460 mg
	Flaxseed	30–60g/day (ground)	$0.31 / 30 gram
	Hypericin	5.6 – 11 mg per day	$0.50 / 6.6 mg

Table 20: Illustration of Compound Costs[96]

Choice	Compound	Research Indicated Range	Example dose cost / day
2 of 4	Apigenin	0.1 – 1.5 g per day	
	Luteolin	0.17 – 1.8 g per day	$2.00 (200mg)
	Genistein	0.1 – 1.1 g per day	
	Quercetin	0.25 – 1.8 g per day	$0.18 (500mg)
1 of 2	Arctigenin	0.65 g per day	
	Arctium seed	12 g per day	$0.86 (12.g)
1 of 2	Boswellic acid	1.8 g per day	$0.98 (1.8 g)
	Asiatic acid	1.7 g per day	
1 of 1	CAPE (Bee propolis)	3 – 15 g per day	$1.50 (10g)
1 of 1	Curcumin	1.5 – 1.8 g per day	$0.62 (1.5g)
1 of 1	Emodin	0.16 – 0.81 g per day	$1.60 (160mg)
1 of 1	EPA/DHA	6 – 21 g per day	$0.33 (6g)
0 or 1	Garlic	6 – 15 g per day	$0.64 (6g)
1 of 3	Limonene	7.3 – 14 g per day	$3.14 (7.3)
	Perillyl alcohol	1.3 – 9 g per day	
	Geraniol	0.27 – 5.7 g per day	
1 of 1	Parthenolide	17 mg per day	$0.65 (17mg)
1 of 1	Resveratrol	68 – 410 mg per day	$0 (with emodin)
1 of 1	Selenium	250 – 1100 µg per day	$0.15 (400µg)
1 of 1	Vitamin A emulsified	50000 – 600000 i.u/day	$0.08 (50000iu)
1 of 1	Vitamin (1,25-D3)	0.75 – 2.5 µg per day	$1.86 (0.75µg)
1 of 2	Vitamin E	440 – 1700 i.u per day	
	Vitamin E succinate	440 – 1700 i.u per day	$0.25 (800iu)
1 of 2	Anthocyanidins	0.12 – 1.8 g per day	
	Proanthocyanidins	0.49 – 1.8 g per day	
1 of 2	Ruscogenins	100 – 130 mg per day	$1.40 (40mg)
	Aesin extract	150 mg per day	
0 or 1	Vitamin C	1 – 2 g per day	$0.15 (2g)
1 of 1	Bromelain	1 – 4 g per day	$1.05 (3.5g)
1 of 1	Astragalus	Include in PSP/PSK grp	$1.50 (=30g)
1 of 2	Siberian Ginseng	Include in PSP/PSK grp	$0.33 (=12g)
	Ginsenoside	110–340mg /day	
1 of 3	PSP/PSK		$1.50 (3g)
	Ganoderma	2 – 9 g of polysaccharides per day	$0.90 (1.9g)
	Shiitake		$0.60 (450mg)
1 of 1	Melatonin	3 – 20 mg per day	$0.35 (10mg)
0 or 1	Glutamine	8-30 mg per day	$1.76 (8g)
0 of 3	EGCG	0.46 – 0.55 g per day	$0.68 (460mg)
	Flaxseed	30–60g/day (ground up)	
	Hypericin	5.6 – 11 mg per day	
Total			$25.06

Table 21: Illustration of Possible Protocol Along With Costs[97]

Compound	Example location for purchase
Apigenin	www.iherb.com/neurodef.html
Luteolin	www.lutimax.com/order.html
Genistein	www.lef.org/newshop/items/item00383.html
Quercetin	www.lef.org/newshop/items/item00470.html
Arctigenin	No supplier of standardised extract yet available
Arctium seed	www.kingherb.com/
Boswellic acid	www.iherb.com/boswellic.html
Asiatic acid	http://secure-shopping-cart.com/niam/cart/cart3.html
CAPE	www.iherb.com/propolis2.html
Curcumin	www.lef.org/newshop/items/item00552.html
Emodin	www.netriceuticals.com/listing.asp?id=390
EPA/DHA	www.lef.org/prod_desc/item00048.html
Garlic	www.vitacost.com/
Limonene	www.iherb.com/pwrdlimonene.html
Perillyl alcohol	www.neways.com/
Geraniol	www.viable-herbal.com/singles/herbs/s826.htm
Parthenolide	http://herbalremedies.com/fevstd60cap.html
Resveratrol	www.netriceuticals.com/
Selenium	www.lef.org
Vit. A emulsified	www.lef.org/newshop/items/item00294.html
Vit. D3 (1,25-D3)	www.realfastdrugstore.com/
Vitamin E	www.lef.org/newshop/category/category32000-p7.html
Vit. E succinate	www.lef.org/prod_desc/item00063.html
Anthocyanidins	www.myvitanet.com/bilcaphealey.html
Proanthocyanidins	http://store.yahoo.com/iherb/grapeseed8.html
Ruscogenins	CircuMax - www.koshervitamin.com
Aesin extract	CircuMax - www.koshervitamin.com
Vitamin C	www.lef.org/newshop/items/item00081.html
Bromelain	Ultra Bromelain 1500mg - www.lef.org
Astragalus	http://store.yahoo.com/iherb/astragalus7.html
Siberian ginseng	http://store.yahoo.com/iherb/ginseng1.html
Panax ginseng	http://store.yahoo.com/iherb/panaxredgin.html
PSP/PSK	http://store.yahoo.com/iherb/coriolus.html
Ganoderma	www.herbalremedies.com/62700.html
Shiitake	http://store.yahoo.com/iherb/shiitake2.html
Melatonin	www.lef.org/newshop/items/item00331.html
Glutamine	www.lef.org/newshop/items/item00345.html
EGCG	www.lef.org/prod_desc/item00444.html
Flaxseed	www.howeseeds.com/
Hypericin	http://store.yahoo.com/iherb/sjwsn.html

Table 22: Example Suppliers for Each Natural Compound[98]

E

Appendix E:
Liver Cleanse Protocol

Ingredients:

4 tablespoons of oral Epsom salts

fi cup virgin olive oil

1 large fresh grapefruit

2 glass jars with lids

16 oz. apple juice + beet juice

First day:

- ❖ **09:00:** Eat a breakfast of cooked porridge, no milk or butter; eight ounces apple juice + beet juice; baked potato, no butter

- ❖ **14:00:** Mix four tablespoons of oral Epsom salts in three cups of cold water in one jar, and refrigerate

- ❖ **15:00:** Have an enema

- ❖ **18:00:** Drink ⁶ cup of the cold Epsom salts

- ❖ **20:00:** Drink ⁶ cup Epsom salts

- ❖ **21:45:** Pour ⁵ cup olive oil into the second jar; squeeze out ⁵ cup grapefruit juice and add to the olive oil. Close the jar lid and shake hard until watery.

- ❖ **22:00:** Drink the potion. Lie down immediately. Lie still on your back and go to sleep.

Second day:

- ❖ **09:00:** Drink ⁶ cup Epsom salts. Go back to bed.

- ❖ **11:00:** Drink ⁶ cup Epsom salts. Go back to bed.

- ❖ **13:00:** Get up and drink eight ounces apple + beet juice.

- ❖ **14:00:** Eat a banana or an orange

- ❖ **18:00:** Eat a light supper of salad and fruit; no meat

Stones [may] be seen in the toilet upon the first bowel movement after a liver cleanse. It may take several cleanses over a period of months to clear all of them out from the liver.

Following a liver cleanse, it is useful to have several coffee enemas to pull further toxins that are stored in the liver.

[Source: http://groups.yahoo.com/group/ozonetherapy/message/1391]

For similar recipes, remarkable photos of stones that are excreted and everything else you want to know about liver cleanses see:

http://curezone.com/cleanse/liver

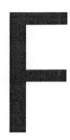

Appendix F: How To Carry Out A Coffee Enema

Note: Do not carry out a coffee enema if you have an allergy to coffee.

Coffee enemas are recommended by many experienced practitioners to help the body detoxify itself of waste substances. We will look at the main ways coffee enemas help—and also outline the procedure to carry out an enema.

Relaxation of muscles

Three chemicals in coffee—caffeine, theophylline and theobromine, encourage muscles to relax and hence cause blood vessels and bile ducts in the liver to dilate. The above three chemicals are far more easily absorbed through the colon compared to the absorbtion rate when coffee is drunk.

Benefits to the liver

Coffee contains enzymes called palmitates—and these help the liver eliminate toxic substances via bile. Because the bile ducts dilate as described above, the bile is able to flow into the gastro-intestinal where it can be later evacuated as part of the enema.

We should note the coffee reaches the liver from the colon because it is first absorbed into the hemorrhoidal vein and then taken up to the liver by the portal vein.

Peristaltic activity of colon

Peristaltic action refers to the contractions of the colon—and these are stimulated by the presence of the extra fluid introduced into the colon by the enema. Towards the end of the enema you will allow the peristaltic contractions of the colon to push waste and toxins out from the body.

Supplies

A low cost reusable enema kit—available from many internet sources.

Luke warm bottled / distilled water—no tap water because it will likely contain chlorine and other substances you will want to keep out of your colon.

Organic coffee—any level of 'roasting' is fine—pre-ground is easier.

Cafetier type coffee maker—(large glass container with press down filter)—or alternatively you can use a saucepan and then filter it.

How to prepare the coffee

- Boil eight cups of water.
- Put eight ground spoons of coffee into the cafetier or pan
- Pour the boiling water onto the ground coffee in the pan or the cafetier and leave for an hour.

- After an hour, check the temperature of the water is around body temperature. If not—do not use until it is body temperature.

- Press the plunger of the cafetier down—so that all the coffee grains are taken out of the fluid (alternatively filter the water through a sieve)—and pour coffee solution into enema bag.

Directions for carrying enema

- Hang the enema bag a foot or so above the height you are going to lie. Then lie on your back or right side—and use the enema tube to 'infuse' the coffee solution into your colon.

- You will probably need to infuse just a little coffee at a time, and the enema kit will likely have a simple 'tube clamp' so you can stop the flow at any time.

- Try and retain the coffee for as long as possible—10-20 minutes is fine.

- As the coffee infuses into your colon, you will feel the fluid in your colon—you can massage your colon starting on your left side and working up until you are just below your navel—then move horizontally across and down your right side.

Concerns

Some people are concerned that using enemas will damage their colon muscles and/or make the muscles lazy. However, this is not correct—rather enemas carried out at appropriate intervals will actually retrain and strengthen the muscles in their peristaltic action.

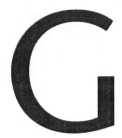

Appendix G: NCI Cantron Test Data

The following table is a summary of the raw test results. Please see - www.healing-cancer.co.uk/resources for a copy of the raw results data as provided by the NCI.

Reductions in Percentage Growth from NCI Test Results

Tumor Type	Perillyl	Taxol	Cancell	Tumor Type	Perillyl	Taxol	Cancell
Leukemia				CNS Cancer			
CCRF-CEM	94	NT	-3	SF-268	85	-44	-84
HL-60 (TB)	85	-25	-63	SF-295	54	NT	-95
K-562	71	-100	-12	SF-539	62	1	NT
MOLT-4	59	0	-12	SNB-19	61	-82	-90
RPMI-8226	63	-39	-21	SNB-75	58	-4	-80
SR	52	1	-33	SNB-78	NT	NT	-37
Non-Small Cell Lung Cancer				U251	70	-85	-99
A549/ATCC	87	1	-49	Melanoma			
ERVX	51	6	NT	LOX IMVI	97	-40	-98
HOP-18	NT	NT	-45	MALME-3M	81	1	-58
HOP-62	70	-17	-80	M14	87	-100	-98
HOP-92	57	20	-52	M19-MEL	NT	NT	-86
NCI-H226	83	-70	-51	SK-MEL-2	91	-52	-33
NCI-H23	53	-38	NT	SK-MEL-28	101	0	-50
NCI-H322M	76	-9	-100	SK-MEL-5	74	NT	-96
NCI-H460	92	-98	-72	UACC-257	92	1	-91
NCI-H522	89	-100	-86	UACC-62	65	-68	-99
LXFL 529	NT	NT	-96	Ovarian Cancer			
Small Cell Lung Cancer				IGROV1	96	2	-41
DMS 114	NT	NT	-86	OVCAR-3	81	-100	-100
DMS 273	NT	NT	-68	OVCAR-4	97	1	-95
Colon Cancer				OVCAR-5	90	2	-100
COLO 205	96	-100	-98	OVCAR-8	78	-97	-82
HCC-2998	75	NT	-68	SK-OV-3	96	6	-46
DLD-1	NT	NT	-38	Renal Cancer			
RCC-898	NT	NT	-68	786-0	75	NT	-100
HCT-116	77	-100	-99	A498	54	2	-86
HCT-15	75	24	-89	ACHN	96	-14	-82
HT29	95	-100	-59	CAKI-1	97	7	-22
KM12	103	2	-89	RXF 393	76	-55	-98
KM20L2	NT	NT	-70	RFX-631	NT	NT	-29
SW-620	NT	0	-80	SN12C	74	-86	-98
				TK-10	113	6	-100
				UO-31	74	57	-90

Table 23: Summary of the
NCI Cantron test data[99]

Notes

[1] Prognostic factors for myasthenia gravis treated by thymectomy: review of 61 cases. Ann Thorac Surg. 1999 Jun;67(6):1568–71.

[2] Transcervical thymectomy for myasthenia gravis achieves results comparable to thymectomy by sternotomy. Ann Thorac Surg. 2002 Aug;74(2):320–6; discussion 326–7.

[3] Thymectomy for Myasthenia Gravis. Curr Treat Options Neurol. 2002 May;4(3):203–209.

References

[1] Anne Frähm & David Frähm, Cancer Battle Plan (Tarcher Putman, 1997)

[2] http://holisticonline.com/Light_Therapy/light_intro.htm

[3] http://www.purefood.org/Organic/UKOrganicStudy.cfm

[4] http://www.wigmore.org/

[5] Spiegel, D., et al. 'Group Support for Patients with Metastatic Cancer', (Archives of General Psychiatry 38:527–33, 1981)

[6] Burton Goldberg, Definitive Guide To Cancer, (Future Medicine Publishing, 1997), p.160

[7] http://hcd2.bupa.co.uk/fact_sheets/html/colonic_cancer.html

[8] www.coffee-enema.co.uk/sawilsons/index.html

[9] www.lef.org/magazine/mag2003/feb2003_report_prevent_01.html

[10] Dr. Jimmy Gutman's, 'Glutathione: The Body's Most Powerful Healing Agent', ebook publication

[11] Duncan Crow – Personal correspondence

[12] Ralph Moss, Cancer Therapy, (Equinox, 1992), p.243

[13] Dr Joanna Budwig, Flax Oil As A True Aid Against Arthritis, Heart Infarction, Cancer & Other Diseases, (Apple Publishing, 1992)

[14] Erasmus, U. 'Fatty Degeneration: Cancer Fats and Oils: The complete Guide to Fats and Oils in Health and Nutrition (Vancouver, Canada: Alive Books, 1988), 303–304.

[15] Oxygen-Ozone Therapy – A Critical Evaluation, Velio Bocci (Kluwer Academic Publishers, 2002), p.76

[16] ibid

[17] Ralph Moss, Cancer Therapy, (Equinox, 1992), p.379

[18] Lee, Sweet & Hagar, Ozone selectively inhibits growth of human cancer cells, Science, Volume 209, August 22, 1980, p.931–932

[19] Ozone As A Modulator Of The Immune System (Alessandra Larini et al)

[20] Nathaniel Altman, Oxygen Healing Therapies, (Healing Arts Press, 1995), p.94

[21] 100% Success in Eradicating M.R.S.A from Wounds & Urinary Bladder using Medical Ozone Treatments – Deb, Fennell & Ostle – 2001

[22] Natural Compounds in Cancer Therapy, John Boik (Oregon Medical Press, 2001), p.2

[23] Natural Compounds in Cancer Therapy, John Boik (Oregon Medical Press, 2001), adapted from table p.7 & table p.157

[24] Natural Compounds in Cancer Therapy, John Boik (Oregon Medical Press, 2001), p.242

[25] http://www.digitalnaturopath.com/treat/T8769.html

[26] Natural Compounds in Cancer Therapy, John Boik (Oregon Medical Press, 2001), p.253

[27] http://www.lef.org/magazine/mag2001/aug2001_report_gongalez_01.html

[28] http://www.elec.gla.ac.uk/groups/opto/Kerr.html)

[29] Immune Essay Test conducted on the 714X product (Effect of 714X on peripheral blood monuclear cells in vitro) – March 1999

[30] Cantron: Its Beneficial Role Against Health Damaging Free Radicals: A study and comprehensive discussion of the antioxidant power of Cantron and related formulas by Jerome Godin

[31] ibid

[32] How Entelev/Cancell Works by James Vincent Sheridan & James Edward Sheridan (1992)

[33] ibid

[34] www.nci.nih.gov/cancertopics/pdq/cam/cancell/HealthProfessional/page4

[35] http://alternativecancer.us/testr.htm

[36] http://scri.ngen.com/abstract05.html

[37] Dr Lechin, Neurocircuitry and Neuroautonomic Disorders – Reviews and Therapeutic Strategies (Karger, 2002) by p.76

[38] http://www.burzynskipatientgroup.org/burdickreport.htm

[39] Ralph Moss, Cancer Therapy, (Equinox, 1992), p.239

[40] ibid, p.238

[41] Patient responses to Cytoluminescent Therapy for cancer: an investigative report of early experiences and adverse effects of an unconventional form of photodynamic therapy. Integr Cancer Ther. 2003 Dec;2(4):371–89

[42] ibid

[43] ibid

[44] ibid

[45] Personal correspondence with Bill Porter

[46] ibid

[47] ibid

[48] ireland.com/newspaper/front/2004/0501/1559013515HM1PORTERNEWS.html

[49] www.hippocratesinst.com

[50] Anne Frähm & David Frähm, Cancer Battle Plan (Tarcher Putman, 1997), p.21

[51] http://www.rationaltherapeutics.com/approach/index.html

[52] Personal correspondence with Rational Therapeutics

[53] Data adapted from Cecils Textbook of Medicine, 18

[54] ibid

[55] ibid

[56] ibid

[57] Sheila Snow and Mali Klein, Essiac: The Secrets of Rene Caisse Herbal Pharmacy (Newleaf, 2001)

[58] Adapted from Sheila Snow and Mali Klein, Essiac: The Secrets of Rene Caisse Herbal Pharmacy (Newleaf, 2001)

[59] I Was Canada's Cancer Nurse – The Story of ESSIAC by Rene M. Caisse

[60] ibid

[61] ibid

[62] ibid

[63] http://www.ompress.com/community-faq-2.htm , John Boik article on Essiac

[64] www.cancer.gov/cancerinfo/pdq/cam/mistletoe/HealthProfessional#Section_55

[65] Ewan Cameron & Linus Pauling, Cancer and Vitamin C, (Camino Books, 1979), p.97

[66] ibid p.94

[67] ibid p.xii

[68] ibid p.144

[69] Ewan Cameron & Linus Pauling, Cancer and Vitamin C, (Camino Books, 1979), p.209

[70] The Prime Cause and Prevention of Cancer (Revised lecture at the meeting of the Nobel-Laureates on June 30, 1966), Otto Warburg

[71] ibid

[72] Dr. Otto Warburg, 'On The Origin of Cancer Cells,' Science, (24 February 1956) Volume 123, Number 3191, pp.309–314

[73] Otto Warburg, The Prime Cause And Prevention Of Cancer, (Konrad Triltsch, 1969)

[74] Ewan Cameron & Linus Pauling, Cancer and Vitamin C, (Camino Books, 1979), p.4

[75] Philip Day, Why We're Still Dying To Know The Truth, (Credence Publications, 1999), p.25

[76] Cancer Chronicles by Ralph Moss, Link Between Trophoblasts & Cancer Corroborated, 1977

[77] The Phase III Gonzalez Protocol Trial – http://www.cancer.gov/clinical_trials/doc.aspx?viewid=B7014C36-50A1-4464-B28B-7C5DF89EAA5A

[78] Philip Day, B17 Metabolic Therapy (Credence Publications, 2002), p.65

[79] Philip Day, Why We're Still Dying To Know The Truth, (Credence Publications, 1999), p.110

[80] Ralph Moss, Cancer Therapy, (Equinox, 1992), p.294

[81] ibid p.293

[82] Philip Day, Why We're Still Dying To Know The Truth, (Credence Publications, 1999), p.176

[83] ibid p.127

[84] ibid p.58–59

[85] ibid p.148

[86] Natural Compounds in Cancer Therapy, John Boik (Oregon Medical Press, 2001), adapted from table p.7 & table p.157

[87] ibid

[88] ibid

[89] http://alternativecancer.us/testr.htm

Index